BELLY FAT
BREAKTHROUGH

BELLY FAT
BREAKTHROUGH

Understand What It Is and Lose It Fast

DR. STEPHEN BOUTCHER

GALLERY BOOKS

New York London Toronto Sydney New Delhi

This publication contains the opinions and ideas of its author. It is intended to provide helpful and informative material on the subjects addressed in the publication. It is sold with the understanding that the author and publisher are not engaged in rendering medical, health, or any other kind of personal professional services in the book. The reader should consult his or her medical, health, or other competent professional before adopting any of the suggestions in this book or drawing inferences from it.

The author and publisher specifically disclaim all responsibility for any liability, loss, or risk, personal or otherwise, which is incurred as a consequence, directly or indirectly, of the use and application of any of the contents in this book.

G

Gallery Books
A Division of Simon & Schuster, Inc.
1230 Avenue of the Americas
New York, NY 10020

Copyright © 2014 by Steve Boutcher

First published in 2013 in Great Britain by Nero,
an imprint of Schwartz Media Pty Ltd.

All rights reserved, including the right to reproduce this book
or portions thereof in any form whatsoever. For information
address Gallery Books Subsidiary Rights Department,
1230 Avenue of the Americas, New York, NY 10020

First Gallery Books hardcover edition September 2014

GALLERY BOOKS and colophon are registered trademarks
of Simon & Schuster, Inc.

For information about special discounts for bulk purchases,
please contact Simon & Schuster Special Sales at 1-866-506-1949
or business@simonandschuster.com.

The Simon & Schuster Speakers Bureau can bring authors to your live event. For
more information or to book an event contact the Simon & Schuster Speakers
Bureau at 1-866-248-3049 or visit our website at www.simonspeakers.com.

Cover design by Janet Perr

Manufactured in the United States of America

10 9 8 7 6 5 4 3 2 1

Library of Congress Cataloging-in-Publication Data

Boutcher, Stephen H. (Stephen Hugh), 1949-
Belly fat breakthrough : understand what it is and lose it fast / Steve Boutcher.
pages cm
Includes bibliographical references and index.
ISBN 978-1-4767-7550-0 (alk. paper)
1. Weight loss. 2. Reducing exercises. I. Title.
RM222.2.B646 2014
613.2'5—dc23
2014000233

ISBN 978-1-4767-7550-0
ISBN 978-1-4767-7551-7 (ebook)

I would like to thank the many subjects in our studies who carried out these interval sprinting programs. Thanks also go to the many medical students who made a significant contribution to data collection. A team of PhD students organized and ran these studies, including Mehrdad Heydari, Ehsan Ghareman, and Sarah Dunn. The team at Black Inc. provided invaluable help that made this book possible. Finally, I would like to thank my wife, Yati, who made a significant contribution to the book, both from her published studies and with her editorial help and suggestions.

Contents

Introduction

The human body is programmed to store fat for a number of reasons, but the places it stores fat have different effects on our health. Fat under the skin on our legs and arms is considered a healthy fat and helps to prevent diseases such as type 2 diabetes. In contrast, visceral fat, or belly fat, clusters around our internal organs and has been found to contribute to the development of diabetes and cardiovascular and other inflammatory diseases. This is because the fat in the belly is released to the liver, which affects the way our body reacts to insulin, a hormone produced by the pancreas. Insulin carries the sugar in the blood to the cells of the body, for use as energy. Excessive belly fat eventually brings about decreased insulin sensitivity, potentially causing type 2 diabetes and leading to other serious diseases.

Factors such as age, gender, genes, and lifestyle all influence the amount of fat that is deposited around the organs in your belly. For example, women who are past childbearing age, or postmenopausal, typically have greater belly fat stores than younger women. Similarly, older men tend to have more belly fat than young men do. It has also been discovered that people of Asian descent who experience increases in belly fat have a greater incidence of cardiovascular problems than non-Asians. People who are under stress and those who sleep poorly also tend to have more belly fat. And, of course, individuals who consume a lot of junk food and excessive alcohol and do little exercise typically possess greater belly fat stores.

Our research in the School of Medical Sciences at the University of New South Wales has found that an interval sprinting program, combined with a healthy Mediterranean eating plan, is the most effective way to reduce dangerous belly fat. Interval sprinting involves short bursts of intensive exercise followed by a brief period of light exercise, repeated continuously for twenty minutes. The program we developed has been scientifically shown to improve overall health in much less time than conventional exercise programs such as jogging and weight training. Our interval sprinting program recommends exercising for twenty minutes a session, three times per week—a total of about one hour of exercise a week. By exercising for only one hour a week, you can reduce your belly and body fat, as well as increase the muscle mass in your legs and abdomen, which is important for preventing type 2 diabetes. Interval sprinting has also been proved to significantly reduce insulin resistance—the key for long-term health—and improve cardiovascular health within just six weeks.

Combining the interval sprinting program with a healthy Mediterranean eating plan can extend the health benefits of interval sprinting. Of course, if you begin an exercise program but continue to eat in an unhealthy manner, you'll be undermining the positive effects of the exercise.

Eating healthy foods and participating in a well-structured interval sprinting program can significantly reduce your belly fat and improve your health. This book will show you how.

How to Use This Book

This book contains:

- the interval sprinting program to help you lose belly fat, increase aerobic fitness and muscle mass, and reduce insulin resistance;

- information about healthy eating and which nutrients to ingest before and after sprinting exercise for the best results; and

- a guide to reducing the effect of daily stressors and enhancing sleep quality to prevent an increase in belly fat.

Chapter 1 explains why belly fat is so dangerous to ongoing good health, how it accumulates, and how to determine whether you are carrying a dangerous amount of belly fat. Chapter 2 describes the biological mechanisms by which interval sprinting can help reduce belly fat and increase your overall health. Chapter 3 covers the types of exercises suited to interval sprinting and the program itself. Chapters 4 and 5 show you how to apply the exercise, healthy eating, and stress-management programs to your life. Finally, chapter 6 offers a sample plan for incorporating the *Belly Fat Breakthrough* into your life.

Chapter 1
Understanding Belly Fat

Americans are getting fatter and more obese. Two thirds of adults (66 percent) are currently overweight or obese.[2] A third of adults (36 percent) are currently overweight. This is true in a majority of the developed world, such as Australia and Europe. Australia now has the second highest rate of childhood obesity, while in the United Kingdom, the number of obese adults increased from 16 percent to 24 percent among women and from 13 percent to 22 percent among men between 1993 and 2009. There is also potential for a dramatic increase in obesity rates in India, the Middle East, Asia, and other developing areas, as overweight and obesity rates there have escalated since the 1990s.[2]

We're also seeing a rise in dangerous belly fat, as demonstrated by the increase in average waist circumferences around the world. Having a waist circumference less than 31 inches for women and 37 inches for men is recommended for health reasons, but in the United States, the average waist circumference went from 35 inches in 1962 to 39 inches in 2000 in men, and from 30 inches to 37 inches in women.[3] Another US study monitored more than one hundred thousand middle-aged men and women over nine years. Results showed that people with large waists—greater than 47 inches for men and 43 inches for women—were twice as likely to die prematurely as those with normal waist sizes.[4] In the United Kingdom, a 2011 study found that the average waist circumference of young girls, 28 inches, was 5 inches bigger than girls of the same age measured thirty years previously.[5]

As world levels of belly fat increase, so does the incidence of both type 2 diabetes and cardiovascular disease, so it's important that we understand why we are putting on belly fat and how we can stop this trend.

The Skinny on Fat

We have a layer of fat under the skin called subcutaneous fat. This fat makes up about 80 percent to 90 percent of our total body fat and is typically located on the back of the arms, below the shoulder blades, around the belly, and on the upper legs and hips. The remaining 10 percent to 20 percent of our body fat is termed belly fat, also known as visceral fat, and is located beneath the stomach muscles and around internal organs such as the liver, spleen, intestines, and kidneys. In some people, belly fat can also accumulate in the liver and other organs. Interestingly, people with more fat on their upper thighs have less incidence of type 2 diabetes and cardiovascular disease.[6]

Subcutaneous fat serves a number of purposes, such as

keeping us warm and acting as a storage site for hormones and energy. Also called adipose tissue, it used to be considered mainly a ready source of energy in times of famine, but fat is now viewed as an endocrine organ that stores and excretes a number of hormones and other chemicals that can have both positive and negative effects on health. Endocrine refers to cells, glands, and tissues that secrete hormones into the bloodstream to control our physiology and behavior. Fat mass secretes over thirty chemical messengers; some of them, such as the hormone leptin, tell the brain that we have had enough to eat, whereas others, like tumor necrosis factor, induce inflammation to help combat bacteria, viruses, and other disease-producing pathogens.

Too much inflammation, however, results in cardiovascular disease and insulin resistance. The latter condition occurs when the muscle and liver cells become unresponsive to insulin in the blood. High levels of insulin and glucose remaining in the circulation increase the risk of type 2 diabetes. People with type 2 diabetes typically have excessive belly fat, chronic high blood pressure, or hypertension, and elevated blood triglyceride levels. Fat cells also secrete a chemical called adiponectin, which has antidiabetic properties. Unfortunately, obese people have less of this beneficial chemical.

We all possess billions of fat cells, but it has been shown that an absolute fat cell number is established during the teenage years, and this remains constant during adulthood. One study that assessed genomic DNA was able to retrospectively measure fat cell numbers in humans.[7] A genome is a body's total set of DNA and includes all its genes. Each genome contains all the information needed to create and maintain a human body. Both obese and lean children established their peak fat cell numbers during adolescence, with little change occurring during adulthood. Importantly, those who became obese during adolescence possessed billions more fat cells than their leaner counterparts. As the fat cell lasts about eight to ten years before dying, a natural process known as apoptosis, any extra fat cells that children develop increase their fat-storage capacity, which leads to obesity, and overweight teenagers will therefore have those billions of extra fat cells for the rest of their lives.

Belly fat is different from subcutaneous fat and is much more dangerous, as it contributes to type 2 diabetes and cardiovascular and inflammatory diseases.[8] As can be seen in figure 1, belly fat lies underneath the tummy muscles. Because belly fat is firmer than subcutaneous fat, it pushes the abdominal muscles outward. These fat cells, residing deep in the abdomen, do not release their free fatty acids into the bloodstream but deliver them straight to the liver. In response, the liver produces other forms of fat, called triglyceride and cholesterol, which are then secreted into the circulation. When fat in a fat cell is broken down and transported into your blood, it is referred to as free fatty acid, whereas triglyceride is also a type of fat found in the blood and is used by the body for energy. High triglyceride and cholesterol levels are associated with increased risk of cardiovascular disease.

Belly fat cells also have a greater blood supply than subcutaneous fat cells do, and thus can release fatty acids and hormones far more quickly. The good news is that, compared with subcutaneous fat cells, belly fat cells are far more responsive to circulating catecholamines. These are the major hormones for promoting fat release and fat burning, and they can be significantly elevated by interval sprinting exercise, as discussed in chapter 3. This means that belly fat is easier to lose than subcutaneous fat.

How Belly Fat Accumulates

Belly fat accumulation is influenced by a number of factors, such as possessing high levels of fat-storing hormones and low levels of fat-burning hormones; being sedentary; and having a genetic predisposition to developing belly fat. Eating too much processed food is also related to increases in belly fat and is covered in more detail in chapter 4. Other factors affecting belly fat development accumulation include age, ethnicity, and lifestyle.

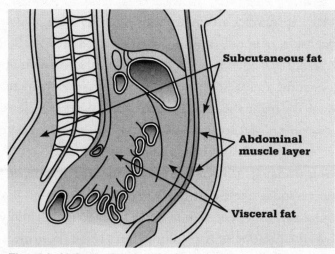

Figure 1. Abdominal stores of subcutaneous and belly fat (visceral fat)

Fat-Storing Hormones

Cortisol, a hormone that is secreted into the blood by the adrenal gland atop each kidney, is typically elevated during moments of stress. When blood cortisol levels increase, the amount of sugar in the blood also increases, which results in a corresponding rise in insulin. Having elevated levels of cortisol and insulin in the blood encourages fat storage and impedes fat burning. This means that high levels of stress increase the concentrations of the two hormones, leading to reduced fat release and increased belly fat stores. Cortisol may also contribute to leptin resistance, which means that people eat more, since fat cells discharge the satiety hormone to tell the brain we are full.

Fat-Burning Hormones

The catecholamines are epinephrine (or adrenaline) and norepinephrine (or noradrenaline) and are secreted into the blood by the adrenal glands. Norepinephrine is also released at nerve endings. Blood catecholamine levels gradually increase through the night and typically peak around eleven o'clock in the morning. Catecholamine-induced fat mobilization occurs much more in belly fat than in subcutaneous fat.

Unfortunately, this catecholamine-induced release of fat is suppressed in obese individuals. This suppression occurs at a young age, as it is present in obese teenagers and children, whose mobilization of triglyceride stores by epinephrine was decreased by 30 percent during rest. This inability to mobilize lipids increases the amount of fat depots in our bodies and can lead to abdominal obesity. Its cause is undetermined but appears to be influenced by defective fat cell receptors. Receptors are specialized proteins located on the outside of cells that allow communication between the cell and the body. Another fat-burning hormone is growth hormone, which is produced by the brain's pituitary gland. Insulin slows down growth hormone release, so people with high levels of insulin in their blood typically have lower levels of growth hormone. Having problems with the thyroid gland can also result in increased belly fat accumulation. The thyroid, an endocrine gland located at the base of the neck, releases a hormone called T-3 (thyroid hormone), which elevates our metabolic rate. Metabolic rate is the amount of energy expended daily at rest. In addition, together with catecholamines and growth hormone, it prompts cells to release more fat. Hypothyroidism occurs when the thyroid gland produces too little T-3 or cells' T-3 receptors become insensitive. Low thyroid levels can contribute to elevated fat deposition and can cause an increase in belly fat stores, and they are often accompanied by elevated low-grade inflammation, as hypothyroid individuals have been shown to possess increased levels of C-reactive protein, an inflammatory chemical, in their blood.

Genetic Influences

Over the past three decades, researchers have discovered genetic markers that contribute to increased body weight and waist circumference; however, no single gene has been found to cause obesity. A genetic marker is an altered gene or DNA sequence that indicates an elevated risk of developing a specific disease or health problem. Specific genes related to obesity have been identified; among them are a number of single-gene mutations that play a part in the development of obesity in teenagers and young adults. This means we now know that genes affect belly fat development when influenced by factors such as physical inactivity, nutrient intake, and metabolic status.

Lifestyle Factors That Influence Belly Fat Accumulation

Many lifestyle factors impact belly fat, but perhaps the most important (after diet and exercise) are age, drinking alcohol, ethnicity, smoking, stress, and sleep. Exposure to daily stressors and reduced quality of sleep have both been associated with belly fat accumulation. Chapter 5 covers how poor sleep and uncontrolled daily stress can lead to belly fat development, together with a description of stress-management and sleep-enhancing techniques.

PHYSICAL INACTIVITY

People who do not take part in recreational exercise and have little physical activity in their jobs are prone to belly fat accumulation, especially if they consume a lot of processed food. Exercising burns up energy and gradually makes the body metabolize more fat than carbohydrate. Carbohydrates are found in fruits and are broken down by the body to be used as energy. They are also present in unhealthy processed foods such as sugar and white bread. It is also likely that fat burning continues during the period after exercise. See chapter 2 for a discussion of how different forms of exercise have differing effects on body fat and muscle mass.

Genes play a role in aerobic fitness levels, and estimates of their contribution to such fitness vary between 10 percent and 40 percent. If you have parents who were good at activities such as cross-country running, it is likely that you will carry genes that will make you good at performing aerobic running exercise. However, all kinds of fitness are influenced mainly by exercising, and to keep fit, you need to perform physical activity. Medical professionals called exercise physiologists assess people's aerobic fitness by exercising them to exhaustion on a bike or treadmill and measuring their maximum oxygen uptake, which reflects aerobic fitness. Determining maximum oxygen uptake, however, requires expertise and expensive equipment. An easier way of assessing aerobic fitness is to see how far you can walk or run on level ground in twelve minutes. This test, the Cooper Twelve-Minute Walk/Run Fitness Test, is described in appendix A, on page 183. For endnote see 1, page 219.

On page 15 you'll find a questionnaire assessment that does not involve exercising. If you score 9 points or less on the questionnaire, or walk or run less than 0.6 miles on the walk/run fitness test, it is likely that you are really unfit and need to begin a fitness program.

AGE

Older people tend to have more belly fat than young people. The main reason for this seems to be a decrease in the body's metabolism: after the age of thirty, most people's metabolism diminishes about 1 percent every two years. Why metabolism slows down as we age is unclear, but it probably involves a decrease in muscle mass and a change in hormone levels. While the amount of subcutaneous fat generally declines with aging, so does muscle mass, and since skeletal muscles, together with the liver, are the major fat-burning engines of the body, older people burn lower levels of fat overall.

The decrease in muscle mass with aging, however, is not inevitable, as people who perform regular weight training typically retain most of their muscle mass and ability to lift weights. Thus, most people see their muscle mass deteriorate as they grow older simply because they are not challenging their skeletal muscles regularly. The good news is that interval sprinting exercise can significantly increase muscle mass.

As we age, blood hormone levels can decrease because of reduced secretion by the body's endocrine glands. The receptors on the body's cells can become insensitive and don't respond to hormones effectively. For women, the largest hormonal change concerns reduced estrogen production when they enter menopause, whereas for men, the largest hormonal change typically involves reduced testosterone.

ALCOHOL

Alcohol contains 7 calories per gram, which is more than the 4 calories contained in a gram of carbohydrate and protein and just under the 9 calories per gram of dietary fat. A calorie is a unit of energy and refers to energy consumption

Answer the questions with regard to your typical weekly physical activity patterns. Fill in a score of 1 to 4 for each question and then add up your total.

1 = Not at all   2 = Sometimes

3 = Fairly regularly   4 = All the time

1. I exercise (walk, run, cycle, swim)
    at least three times per week

2. My exercise sessions last for at
    least thirty minutes

3. When I exercise I breathe
    heavily and sweat

4. My daily job involves a lot of
    physical activity

5. I do a lot of housework
    and gardening

6. During my recreation time, I do a
    lot of physical activity

TOTAL

Interpreting your score:

6 to 9 points: low levels of physical activity

10 to 12 points: moderately low levels of physical activity

13 to 18 points: moderately high levels of physical activity

19 to 24 points: high levels of physical activity

generated by eating, drinking, and physical activity. Thus, consuming two to three average-sized alcoholic drinks a day adds up to over 500 calories. In a week, over 3,500 extra calories would be consumed. Since 1 gram of fat equals 9 calories, that means having three drinks every day of the week adds almost 400 grams of fat to your diet. According to studies in this area, the majority of these calories appear to be deposited as belly fat. It has also been shown that drinking alcohol makes people hungry.

However, a small amount of daily beer or wine, containing 14 grams of ethanol for women and about 28 grams for men, is beneficial for health. An average drink—a regular-sized glass of beer or wine—contains about 14 grams of ethanol, the inebriating agent in alcohol. Studies have shown that women who imbibe about one drink a day and men who consume two drinks a day have a lower incidence of diabetes, stroke, and heart disease.[9]

ETHNICITY

Surprising differences emerge when belly fat accumulation is compared among different ethnicities. Louisiana State University researchers found similar results to a number of other studies showing that African American women possessed less belly fat compared with Caucasian women.[10] A US-Canadian research study of African American and Caucasian men had similar findings.[11] An article published in the *International Journal of Obesity* also indicated that Japanese American men had greater amounts of belly fat than Caucasian men.[12]

However, the strongest relationship between belly fat accumulation and negative health consequences seems to be found in people of South Asian descent. Research conducted at the State University of New York Downstate Medical Center found high amounts of belly fat in Indian migrants, although they were not obese.[13] And according to a 2011 study by Canadian researchers, men and women of South Asian descent accumulated dangerous belly fat on and in their internal organs when they put on total body fat. In contrast, people of Caucasian descent added fat to their waistlines rather than deep inside their bellies.[14] These researchers also discovered that people originally from India, even though they possessed a similar body mass index (BMI) as Caucasians did, had significantly more belly fat. They also had more cardiovascular disease risk factors such as metabolic syndrome and high cholesterol. Metabolic syndrome is a medical name for a number of risk factors that increase the risk for heart disease, stroke, and type 2 diabetes. The researchers suggested that, compared with people of Caucasian descent, those of South Asian heritage had less room beneath their skin to store fat (subcutaneous fat); therefore, their excess fat was stockpiled in fat compartments deep in the belly.

Overall, the increase in belly fat appears to be particularly troublesome in people of South Asian descent, as it seems to give rise to more health problems, such as atherosclerosis and type 2 diabetes. This is why the BMI cutoff for health problems caused by being overweight sometimes differs by ethnicities. (See table 1, page 22.)

Why small increases in belly fat in people of Asian descent

bring about greater cardiovascular problems than in non-Asians is unclear. Why people with South Asian heritage are getting fatter, however, is likely due to a change in lifestyle. People of Asian ethnicity compared with those from Europe have typically possessed far less body and belly obesity, due to their plant-based diets and physically active lifestyles. However, developing countries such as India and China are now adopting Westernized habits that involve consuming much more processed food and performing far less physical activity. The outcome is that countries that used to have very low levels of obesity and type 2 diabetes now have the fastest growth rates of these medical conditions.

SMOKING

Typically, smokers weigh less than nonsmokers, as smoking may reduce appetite and also elevate metabolic rate, which induces fat burning. There is evidence, however, to show that cigarette smoking increases belly fat accumulation: a large, population-based study in the United Kingdom found that men and women who smoked possessed increased belly fat.[15] How smoking increases belly fat is unclear, but shortly after a smoker finishes a cigarette, blood cortisol levels can increase for up to thirty minutes. We know that cortisol can increase belly fat accumulation due to its effect on blood sugar and insulin levels. Smokers also exercise far less than nonsmokers, which is also likely to contribute to increased belly fat accumulation.

The Impact of Belly Fat on Health

Increased belly fat has been associated with the following medical conditions:

- cardiovascular disease

- type 2 diabetes

- hypertension

- elevated blood cholesterol

- increased blood sugar

- dementia

- asthma

- colorectal cancer

- breast cancer

- pancreatic cancer

- endometriosis

- gallbladder disorders

- sleep apnea

For example, in Chinese adults, a bigger waist circumference—an indicator of belly fat—predicted development of hypertension, regardless of whether a person was normal weight or overweight.[16] Another study found that older people with more belly fat had poorer memories and were less verbally fluent.[17]

Interestingly, researchers from Spain tracked 3,235 adult men and women for two years and found that waist circumference predicted disability. People with the largest waist circumference had 2.2 times more risk of mobility disability and 4.8 times more agility disability compared with adults with lower waist circumference.[18] And in a European study of nearly a half million women, excessive belly fat, estimated by waist-to-hip ratio, was related to heightened colorectal cancer risk.[19]

Possessing elevated levels of body and belly fat increases general cancer risk, and people with large waistlines are at higher risk for developing bowel, breast, and pancreatic cancers, and, in postmenopausal women, for cancer of the womb lining, or endometrium. Studies have also shown that in both young and older Japanese American men, belly fat obesity predicted heart attack and hypertension development. Belly fat accumulation has also been associated with gallstones and Alzheimer's disease.

How to Measure Your Body Fat and Belly Fat

Measuring body fat accurately is difficult. To measure body fat, medical professionals and researchers use methods that include magnetic resonance imaging (MRI), dual-energy X-ray absorptiometry (DEXA), computed tomography (CT scan), underwater weighing, skinfold measurements, Bod Pod (a volume-measuring device), and bioelectrical impedance (opposition to the flow of an electrical current through the body). Unfortunately, most of these methods are expensive, and DEXA and computed tomography expose patients to ionizing radiation. Ionizing radiation refers to radiation that has X-rays or gamma rays. Low-cost indirect measures, such as body mass index (BMI), provide an estimate of body fat.

BMI

BMI is calculated by (1) dividing a person's body weight in pounds by (2) his or her height in inches squared (multiplied by itself), and then (3) multiplying by 703. BMI has been used to identify individuals whose weight increases their risk for heart disease and diabetes. People with BMIs of 25.0 to 29.9 are considered overweight, and those with BMIs of 30.0 or higher are considered obese. However, BMI can be misleading because it does not take into account muscle mass, so very muscular or tall individuals can have a BMI of over 30 but actually be very lean. To calculate your BMI, go to the website of the National Heart, Lung, and Blood Institute (www.nhlbi.nih.gov/guidelines/obesity/BMI/bmicalc.htm) or follow the formula below.

HOW TO CALCULATE YOUR BMI

1.   Divide your weight in pounds by your height in inches squared. For example, a six-foot-tall male weighing 200 pounds would first multiply 72 (inches) by 72, which equals 5,184.

2.   Divide 200 by 5,184.

3.   Multiply that figure (0.0385) by 703 to arrive at a BMI of 27.

Dr. Stephen Boutcher

As can be seen in table 1, a BMI of greater than 25 is considered overweight, whereas a body mass index of 30 or higher is obese. BMI values are independent of age for adults, and although BMI is the same for both genders, it varies according to ethnicity. Evidence from a number of large studies supports a higher mortality risk for Americans possessing a high BMI. In contrast, other studies have shown reductions in mortality risk for obese people. This relationship has been termed the obesity paradox but only appears in certain clinical populations such as those with heart failure and type 2 diabetes and the elderly.

Body Mass Index	Weight Classification
Less than 18.5	Underweight
Less than 16.0	Severe thinness
16.0 to 16.9	Moderate thinness
17.0 to 18.5	Mild thinness
18.5 to 24.9	Normal range
25.0 to 29.9	Pre-obese
30.0 or greater	Obese
30.0 to 34.9	Obese class I
35.0 to 39.9	Obese class II
40.0 or greater	Obese class III

Table 1. Criteria for body mass index (BMI) in adults

Adapted from The International Classification of Adult Underweight, Overweight and Obesity According to BMI.[20]

Bioelectrical Impedance Devices

Bioelectrical impedance analysis devices are relatively cheap but tend to underestimate body fat. Although their results are affected by the amount of water found in bodily tissues, if used regularly under standardized conditions—once a week, after fasting in the morning—they will give a reasonable estimate of body fat change. Optimal body fat levels have been suggested to be around 10 percent to 20 percent in men and 20 percent to 25 percent in women.

A new bioelectrical impedance device for measuring belly or visceral fat has recently been developed by Tanita and is called the Viscan AB-140. Comparisons between this device and estimates of central fat carried out by DEXA have shown that their values are very similar. However, comparisons between gold-standard estimates of belly fat such as MRI and computed tomography do not appear to have been carried out.

Risk category	Gender	Waist circumference
Europeans	Men Women	Greater than 37 inches Greater than 31 inches
South Asian	Men Women	Greater than 35 inches Greater than 31 inches
Chinese	Men Women	Greater than 35 inches Greater than 31 inches
Japanese	Men Women	Greater than 35 inches Greater than 31 inches

Table 2. *International Diabetes Federation Criteria for Ethnic or Country-Specific Values for Waist Circumference*

Adapted from Alberti, Zimmet, and Shaw.[21]

Waist Circumference

Waist circumference is an easy measure to obtain and is strongly related to belly fat assessed by medical techniques such as computed tomography. Thus, having a large waist circumference usually indicates significant belly fat. Measure your waist circumference immediately above your navel, keeping the tape level with the top of your right hip bone. Don't pull the tape measure too tight, and you should take shallow breaths as opposed to holding your breath. Having someone else take the measure reduces error, and it is best if two measurements are taken and the average value recorded. Optimal waist circumferences for men and women of Asian and European descent are indicated in table 2, but if you are very large or tall, these values may be inaccurate. Waist circumference greater than these values is associated with increased cardiovascular and metabolic health problems.

Abdominal Width

Belly fat tends to remain in the same position in your abdomen whether you are standing up or lying down. In contrast, abdominal subcutaneous fat—the fat you can pinch around your tummy—will tend to move sideways and downward when you're lying on your back. To test if you have a lot of belly fat, you can compare your abdominal width when you are standing to when you are lying down:

Stand against a wall, making sure to push your spine against it. Place something flat, such as a plastic ruler, across your abdomen, and then use a tape measure or another ruler to measure your abdominal width from the wall to the plastic ruler. Record the distance. Now lie on a flat surface on your back. Place the ruler on your abdomen and measure from floor to ruler with the tape measure. If the measurement does not change much and if you have a large waist circumference (as per the measurements in table 2), then you likely possess a lot of belly fat. If the difference is substantial—even 1 inch—you probably have a significant amount of subcutaneous abdominal fat.

These simple methods are not exact, but they will let you know if interval sprinting is reducing your belly fat over time. If you undertake the program described in chapter 6, measuring abdominal width and waist circumference weekly are good ways to gauge your progress.

Waist Skinfold Measure

An estimate of total body fat can also be achieved by measuring the thickness of skinfolds in different parts of the body. This is done with a device called skinfold calipers, which ascertains the thickness of the skin together with a layer of subcutaneous fat. Formulas have been developed to estimate the total percentage of body fat from calipers measurements; however, their accuracy has been questioned. Like bioelectrical impedance, calipers measurements are best used to estimate subcutaneous fat change over time rather than one single estimate of total body fat.

Skinfold assessment does not estimate belly fat, but it can be used to monitor changes in the subcutaneous fat around your belly. A useful place to take a measurement is the waist skinfold, which is illustrated in figure 2. The waist, or suprailiac, skinfold is located just above the protrusion of the hip bone, known as the iliac crest. It is more accurate if you get someone else to do the measurement for you. It is important that the skinfold is taken in the same position every time; therefore, it's wise to photograph the site with a digital camera.

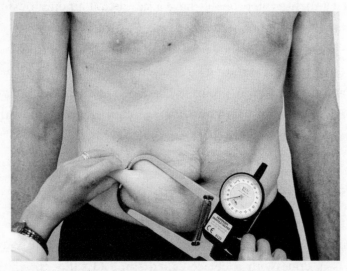

Figure 2. Assessment of waist subcutaneous fat by skinfold

The fold is taken almost horizontally. For right-handed people, pinch and hold a fold of skin with its layer of subcutaneous fat with the left forefinger and thumb. Using the right hand, place the calipers jaws about 0.3 inches from the left forefinger. Keep holding the skinfold with the left hand throughout. Release the calipers so that all the force of the jaws is on the skinfold alone. The calipers will take a few moments to stabilize; the value should be recorded only when they have stopped changing and before releasing any calipers pressure. Measure the waist site twice and record the readings on the Body Composition Recording Form. (See appendix E, page 192.)

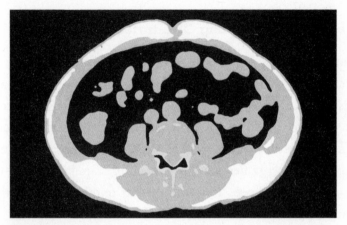

Figure 3. A computed tomography scan across the waist area. White is the subcutaneous abdominal fat, grey is mostly abdominal muscle and other tissue, and black is the belly, or visceral, fat.

*

Now you have three abdominal and belly fat measurements that can be used to monitor subcutaneous and belly fat change as you proceed with the interval sprinting program:

- waist circumference,

- abdominal width, and

- waist skinfold.

If your waist circumference gets smaller, then either your subcutaneous abdominal fat (white) or belly fat (black) has been reduced. If your waist circumference gets smaller but the skinfold calipers measurement does not change, then it is likely that your belly fat has decreased.

How to Measure Leg Circumference

Measuring skeletal muscle mass is best carried out by a medical professional using an imaging procedure such as an MRI or a DEXA. For do-it-yourself monitoring, however, the assessment of leg circumference can provide an indirect guide to possible change in muscle mass after interval sprinting. Leg measurements are obtained in a similar fashion to waist circumference, and are taken at midthigh and at the widest point of the calf.

For the midthigh measurement, use a tape measure to calculate the distance between your groin and the top of your kneecap, and then determine the midpoint of the measurement. You should mark the site with an impermanent ink pen and take a digital picture to ensure that you measure in the same place each time. Stand with your weight evenly distributed on both feet and wrap the tape measure around the midpoint of your thigh. The tape measure should not be pulled too tight. Having someone else take the measurements reduces error, and it is best if two measures are recorded and the average value documented. Write down the results on the Body Composition Recording Form. (See appendix E, page 192.)

*

The key points to remember about the problems of having too much belly fat are:

- Worldwide, belly fat accumulation is increasing dramatically.

- Belly fat increases with a poor diet and physical inactivity.

- Belly fat has a number of negative effects on health.

- Belly fat is influenced by a variety of factors, including diet, inactivity, ethnicity, gender, age, stress, poor sleep, and genetics.

- Belly fat change can be assessed by measuring waist circumference, abdominal width, and waist skinfold, and leg muscle mass change can be assessed by measuring girth circumference.

You should now have an understanding of the differences between belly fat and subcutaneous fat, and of the dangers of carrying high levels of this fat. You might even have identified factors in your own life that can lead to an increase of belly fat and will be able to estimate how much subcutaneous and belly fat you carry. Read on to learn the best ways to combat belly fat and create a healthier life.

Chapter 2
The Effect of Exercise on Belly Fat and Health

Aerobic exercise can result in a loss in belly fat; how-ever, a lot of aerobic exercise has to be performed before you see results. Similarly, carrying out three sessions of resistance exercise per week does not seem to reduce belly fat. In contrast, research has shown that regular interval sprinting will reduce belly fat in far less time than other forms of exercise. In this chapter, you'll find a discussion of the results of published research articles that have examined the effects of aerobic and resistance exercise and interval sprinting on belly fat loss. There is also a discussion of the possible mechanisms that are thought to contribute to the belly fat–reducing effect of interval sprinting and its impact on aerobic fitness, skeletal muscle mass, and insulin resistance.

Aerobic Exercise and Belly Fat

Traditionally, exercise programs to promote fat loss have consisted of steady-state, moderate-intensity activities such as walking, jogging, or swimming for at least forty-five minutes per session. The rationale for this is that individuals burn more fat as fuel during moderate-intensity exercise and should lose more body fat as a result. Disappointingly, many studies have shown that this form of exercise brings about little total body fat loss unless the individual engages in extremely high volumes of aerobic exercise.[1] Likewise, although regular aerobic exercise can affect belly fat loss, you have to do *a lot* of it. For example, researchers at Duke University compared sedentary adults with other volunteers who exercised at light or hard intensity. Results showed that the sedentary people gained about 9 percent of belly fat in six months, whereas adults who walked or jogged about 12.4 miles a week put on no belly fat. Those who jogged only about 18.6 miles a week lost both belly fat and subcutaneous fat, but their muscle mass was unchanged. A greater amount of belly fat (18 percent) was lost by overweight men and women who carried out a fourteen-week aerobic exercise program that involved exercising for sixty-minute sessions five days per week. Again, their muscle mass remained unchanged.

A summary of results of the aerobic exercise studies in this area found that, to reduce belly fat, a person had to work out at least thirty minutes per day—and preferably up to sixty minutes per day—for at least fourteen weeks.[2] Thus, there is evidence to suggest that aerobic exercise for at least forty-five minutes per day, five days per week, for fourteen weeks can produce roughly 18 percent decrease in belly fat without a change in muscle mass. But the reality is that most people do not have the time or the motivation to engage in over five hours of exercise a week; hence the need to find a form of exercise that results in a significant decrease in belly fat while maintaining or increasing muscle mass, and yet is time efficient. Interval sprinting meets all three criteria.

Resistance Exercise and Belly Fat

Strength training, or resistance training—that is, exercising with weights—may also help reduce belly fat accumulation in some individuals. Researchers from the University of Pennsylvania monitored overweight and obese premenopausal women over a two-year period. In comparison to women who did not exercise, participants who performed an hour of weight training twice a week decreased their total body fat by about 4 percent; however, while they did not record an increase in belly fat, the amount of belly fat was not reduced. Two other studies of older men and women demonstrated that three moderately hard weekly weight-training sessions for twelve weeks resulted in little change in total body fat but decreased belly fat substantially. However, far more studies found no effect of resistance exercise on belly fat. A 2012 meta-analysis by one group of researchers reviewed the results of thirty-five well-controlled studies investigating the influence of resistance exercise on belly fat and concluded that it failed to induce significant reductions.[3] A randomized controlled trial is a type of scientific study and is the gold standard in medical research. The key feature of a randomized controlled trial is that subjects to be studied are randomly allocated to receive one or other of the different treatments under examination.

The weight-training protocols used in these studies typically involved around eight different exercises, with eight to ten repetitions apiece, repeated three times each exercise. The individual exercises worked the muscles of the upper arms, the abdomen, and the legs. This type of protocol was generally performed two to three times per week. During a typical sixty-minute weight-training session, the actual time spent lifting weights is about eight to ten minutes. Thus, it is likely that lifting weights at a moderate intensity for eight minutes, three times per week, will not yield significant decreases in body fat or belly fat.

What Is Interval Sprinting?

Interval sprinting protocols typically involve repeated sprinting or hard exercise at near all-out intensity, followed by low-intensity exercise or rest. The length of the sprint period has varied from six seconds to two minutes, and the recovery period has ranged from twelve seconds to four minutes. Most researchers in this area have examined interval sprinting on a stationary cycle ergometer and have studied healthy adolescents, young adults, and older individuals, as well as the following patient groups: (1) those undergoing cardiac rehabilitation, (2) men and women with intermittent claudication (a medical term used to describe muscle pain that occurs during exercise such as walking), (3) type 2 diabetics, and (4) obese children and adults. An ergometer is an exercise machine that measures the amount of work done by human muscles.

One of the most frequently utilized protocols has been

the Wingate test, which consists of thirty seconds of all-out sprint with a hard resistance. Subjects typically perform the Wingate test four to six times, with each sprint being separated by four minutes of recovery. Knowledge about changes to skeletal muscle from interval sprinting has been achieved mainly by using this protocol. However, the Wingate test is extremely challenging, and people have to be highly motivated to tolerate a lot of pain and discomfort. Consequently, the Wingate test is unsuitable for most overweight, sedentary individuals interested in losing belly fat.

Other, less intense interval sprinting protocols have also been applied. For example, we have used an eight-second cycle sprint followed by twelve seconds of low-intensity cycling for a period of twenty minutes. Thus, instead of four to six sprints per session, as used in Wingate studies, participants using the eight-second/twelve-second protocol sprint sixty times at a lower exercise intensity for a total sprint of eight minutes, with twelve minutes of low-intensity cycling. For this method, the total exercise time is twenty minutes, plus a four-minute warm-up and four-minute cool down. Thus, one of the features of interval sprinting is that it takes far less time than traditional aerobic exercise approaches, making it a time-efficient strategy for accruing health benefits.

Interval Sprinting and Belly Fat

Direct measures, such as magnetic resonance imaging, and indirect techniques, like measuring waist circumference, have been used to assess the effects of interval sprinting on belly fat. In one study, French researchers found a 48 percent decrease in belly fat, measured by MRI, after steady-state aerobic exercise two days per week and interval training one day a week for eight weeks in middle-aged men and women.[4] Another investigation of older men, also using MRI, found that eight weeks of aerobic interval training, which also involved vigorous exercise for two minutes and resting for four minutes, resulted in a 14 percent loss of belly fat.

Our research at the University of New South Wales has used a shorter-interval sprinting protocol with younger overweight people. In our first two studies with women, we used DEXA and waist circumference to evaluate belly fat change. DEXA absorptiometry does not assess belly fat directly but does measure a variable called central abdominal fat, which is highly related to belly fat. DEXA absorptiometry scans are used to evaluate bone mineral density but can also measure total body composition and fat content. DEXA absorptiometry uses X-rays to assess bone mineral density but the dose is very low, about one tenth that of a standard chest X-ray. Computed tomography is also a technique used to measure body composition and belly fat but uses a higher radiation dose. Magnetic resonance imaging is another medical imaging technique used in radiology to investigate the anatomy and function of the body. Magnetic resonance imaging scanners use strong magnetic fields and radio waves, thus patients are not exposed to radiation. The first study we conducted lasted fifteen weeks: our subjects undertook twenty minutes of interval sprinting at an eight-second/twelve-second ratio three times per week.[5] They lost 5.7 pounds of total body fat (11 percent), which was accompanied by a significant decrease in central abdominal fat.

In a second study, overweight women exercised for only twelve weeks following the same protocol.[6] They lost 9 percent of total body fat (5.5 pounds) and experienced a 6 percent decrease in central abdominal fat. In this clinical trial, waist circumference was reduced by 1.4 inches after six weeks of interval sprinting. Waist circumference is highly related to central abdominal fat, which suggests that belly fat was significantly reduced after six weeks, or six hours, of interval sprinting. These women also changed their diets to a Mediterranean eating plan, which resulted in a 13 percent decrease in daily caloric intake.

In a third study, we examined a twelve-week interval sprinting program on the belly fat of young overweight men.[7] We measured belly fat with an imaging technique called computed tomography, which uses ionizing radiation to locate the belly fat deep inside the abdomen. Males lost 9 percent of total body fat (4.4 pounds) and 17 percent of belly fat. They also lost 5 percent of subcutaneous abdominal fat. Similar to our studies with women, waist circumference was reduced by 1.4 inches after six weeks of interval sprinting. In the male study, waist circumference was highly correlated with belly fat, suggesting that belly fat was significantly reduced after six weeks, or six hours, of interval sprinting. A summary of the results of studies examining the effects of aerobic exercise, resistance exercise, and interval sprinting on belly fat reduction is shown in table 3.

Because interval sprinting has been studied only relatively recently with subjects who are not athletes, there are fewer published research studies in this area. But it already looks like interval sprinting has led to far greater reductions of total body and belly fat than the other two exercise modalities in significantly less exercise time. It takes just six weeks of interval sprinting exercise to see a substantial reduction in waist circumference, so we can conclude that interval sprinting is the most effective form of exercise for reducing belly fat.

	Interval sprinting	Aerobic exercise	Resistance exercise
Range of total body fat loss	4.4 to 5.5 pounds	2.2 to 3.3 pounds	No change
Range of belly fat percentage loss	17 percent to 48 percent reduction	6 percent to 18 percent reduction	No change
Average waist circumference loss	1.4 inches	0.8 inches	No change
Average hours of exercise	12 hours	70 hours	36 hours

Table 3. Summary of results of randomized, controlled studies examining the effects of aerobic exercise, resistance exercise, and interval sprinting on total fat and belly fat reduction

Adapted from information in studies by Boutcher, Ohkawara, et al., and Ismail et al.[8]

Possible Reasons Why Interval Sprinting Leads to Belly Fat Loss

The mechanisms underlying the interval sprinting–induced belly fat loss include increased exercise and postexercise fat burning, increased muscle mass, decreased appetite after exercise, and reduced postprandial lipemia, which is when triglyceride levels in blood rise after eating. These levels can stay elevated for up to eighteen hours.

Increased Fat Burning

Toward the end of an interval sprinting session involving many repeat sprints, the exercising muscles start to run out of sugar, which, in the form of glucose and glycogen, is needed to create a high-energy compound called adenosine triphosphate. ATP provides the energy for muscular contraction. The body cannot store glucose so it is stored as glycogen. A large amount of glycogen is stored in the liver and skeletal muscles. When interval sprinting decreases the amount of glucose in the body, the stored glycogen is converted to glucose for use by the body. It is believed that toward the end of an interval sprinting session, the ATP is derived mainly from intramuscular fat stores: the fat stockpiled within the skeletal muscles. Together with subcutaneous and belly fat, these depots are an important source of fat. If we don't regularly burn up the fat accumulated in our muscles, insulin resistance and type 2 diabetes usually develop. But when we deplete the fat stores inside the muscle by interval sprinting, the body is forced to replace them with fat stored elsewhere, such as in the belly and under the skin. Furthermore, some of the hormones generated during interval sprinting appear to continue burning fat long after we're finished exercising. Because belly fat is more responsive to interval sprinting, we believe that this shuttling of fat from the belly to the skeletal muscles contributes to long-term reduction of visceral fat stores.

The ability of aerobic exercise to keep burning energy postexercise has been studied extensively. A review of these investigations concluded that a session of aerobic exercise lasting forty minutes or more typically increased energy by about 13 percent. This is a negligible effect likely to make only a small contribution to overall fat loss. The fat-burning response after interval sprinting, however, has not been examined rigorously. It is possible that the high levels of catecholamine in the bloodstream during interval sprinting (see figure 10, page 78) could induce fat burning long after exercise has stopped. This elevation may also happen because of the body's need to lower blood and muscle lactate—a chemical that accumulates during hard exercise—and to resynthesize the depleted glycogen in the exercising muscles. The elevated growth hormone levels documented after a session of interval sprinting may also contribute to enhanced energy expenditure and fat burning.

Increased Muscle Mass

It has been estimated that an increase of 2.2 pounds of skeletal muscle has the capability to burn up about an extra 21 calories per day. In theory, this could amount to just under 6.6 pounds of body fat usage per year. Thus, retaining or increasing muscle mass is very important for health. Unfortunately, it is well documented that aerobic exercise does not change muscle mass, while moderately hard resistance exercise may result in increased muscle mass in some people. A recent review concluded that weight-training programs carried out by middle-aged people yielded an average increase of muscle mass of 2.6 pounds.[9] As can be seen in table 5 (page 51), our three interval sprinting studies demonstrated significant increases of leg and trunk muscle mass of 0.4 pounds and 0.7 pounds for women and 1.1 pounds and 1.5 pounds for men, respectively.[10] Another research group found a large increase in leg muscle mass of older women after they had carried out interval training for sixteen weeks. These results are important, as muscle mass affects health and is typically reduced by aging and when people go on a severe diet.

Decreased Appetite

It is also possible that interval sprinting may help to suppress appetite, which could contribute to belly fat loss. Studies of rats have shown that they eat less after they perform hard exercise. The mechanisms underlying this effect are not known, but strenuous physical exertion may reduce hunger by releasing hormones that curb appetite. For example, corticotropin-releasing factor, a powerful hormone that depresses appetite, has been shown to increase in rats and people during hard running and swimming exercises. Although human studies have shown a large decrease in appetite after intensive aerobic exercise, this effect lasts only for a short time.

The effect of high-intensity sprinting on appetite suppression has been investigated by one study of obese adolescents.[11] Appetite was assessed before and after a six-week high-intensity exercise and diet intervention. The intensive exercise program increased the energy expenditure of the teens; however, their appetites did not increase in line with their energy output. Why individuals do not eat more after hard, intensive exercise is unclear, but animal studies have shown that appetite centers in the brain are affected by blood lactate levels. When people engage in strenuous anaerobic exercise such as interval sprinting, the level of lactate in their bloodstream rises. Anaerobic exercise is brief and quick and involves short exertion, high-intensity movement such as weight lifting, jumping, and sprinting.

Interestingly, in animals, injections of lactate have been shown to suppress appetite. Thus, it is feasible that the increased blood lactate levels brought about by interval sprinting may contribute to suppressing appetite in humans.

Decreased Postprandial Lipemia

Consuming saturated fat or the simple sugar fructose in three meals per day can elevate triglyceride (also called triacylglycerol) levels in the blood for up to eighteen hours. Saturated fat is mainly found in animal products such as meat and foods containing whole milk, whereas simple sugars are glucose found in corn, rice, and wheat products and fructose found in fruit, some vegetables and grains, and honey. This is called postprandial lipemia and is discussed in greater detail in chapter 4. It has been discovered that people with high levels of fat in their blood after eating also tend to have greater belly fat stores. Impressively, just one bout of acute, moderately hard aerobic exercise lasting forty minutes resulted in significantly lower fat in the blood after consumption of a high-fat meal even as long as twelve hours after exercise. Recently, we have shown that interval sprinting has a similar effect. Twenty minutes of interval sprinting at night reduced by about 13 percent the fat (triglyceride) in the blood of young women who ate a high-fat meal the next morning.[12] The mechanism underlying this effect is believed to be the ability of moderately hard exercise to increase an enzyme called lipoprotein lipase, which is located in the muscle capillaries. One of its major roles is to escort triglyceride from the circulation and into the muscles that have been exercised. The increase in lipoprotein lipase usually peaks about four to six hours after physical activity but stays elevated for up to eighteen hours postexercise.

This effect of exercise on lipoprotein lipase may also play a critical role in the belly fat reduction found after interval sprinting. As discussed, the major hormones that induce fat release from belly fat cells are the catecholamines. Interval sprinting, in contrast to moderate aerobic exercise like walking, results in significantly greater blood levels of catecholamines. We have discovered that belly fat is far more sensitive to the effect of catecholamines than are the fat cells beneath the skin, so more fat is released from the belly fat cells during interval sprinting than from other fat stores. However, all belly fat that is released goes directly to the liver via the portal vein, where most of it is repackaged as triglyceride and secreted back into the circulation. So where does this fat in the form of triglyceride go? Although studies have not yet determined the destination, it is feasible that, similar to the elevated triglyceride found after a high-fat meal, the increased circulating triglyceride is shuttled into the skeletal muscle by the increased levels of lipoprotein lipase caused by exercise. This sequence of events is illustrated in figure 4.

How Much Body and Belly Fat Is It Possible to Lose After Interval Sprinting?

The amount of total body fat loss expected to take place after exercise can be assessed by estimating the energy cost of the exercise. For example, the most body fat that an untrained individual can burn during a bout of aerobic cycling has been estimated to be 0.02 ounces per minute. Assuming an optimal fat metabolizing rate of 0.02 ounces per minute for one sixty-minute session of cycling, exercise would result in an energy usage equivalent of about 1.3 ounces of fat. Thus, a twelve-week aerobic exercise program consisting of moderately intense cycling five times a week for sixty minutes each session could theoretically result in a fat mass loss of around 6 pounds, after adding the potential 13 percent more fat burning that may occur postexercise. Over the course of a year, fat loss could total around 28 pounds.

However, as mentioned previously, fat loss from aerobic exercise is usually much less than this amount because of a number of factors, such as compensatory eating and a reduction in other forms of daily physical activity. Also, a range of individual, physiological, and medical factors—among them genetics, fat-burning ability, and thyroid dysfunction—may impede fat loss in certain individuals.[13] In contrast, some people who exercise may lose much greater amounts of body fat, which most likely reflects the fact that they undertook a starvation diet at the same time they started their exercise program. Consequently, the most likely explanation for large increases or decreases in total fat mass after exercise is a change in diet. As we'll see in chapter 4, starvation diets don't work for most people in the long term and are associated with a number of health problems. A reasonable amount of total body fat loss to expect after fifteen weeks of interval sprinting is around 6.6 pounds.

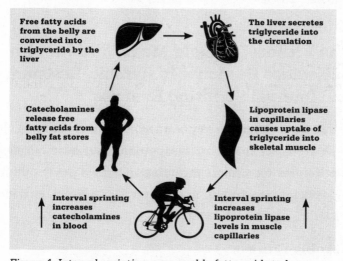

Figure 4. *Interval sprinting may enable fatty acids to be transported from belly fat cells into the liver and then back into the circulation in the form of triglyceride, which is then shuttled into the skeletal muscles.*

The decrease in dangerous belly fat, however, is difficult to estimate, although it is known that belly fat is easier to lose than subcutaneous fat. For example, as mentioned earlier, in the third of our three studies, men lost 17 percent of their belly fat, 9 percent of their total subcutaneous body fat, and 5 percent of their subcutaneous abdominal fat.[14]

Thus, percentagewise, they lost three times more belly fat than abdominal fat after twelve weeks of interval sprinting. Similar to our study with women, the waist circumference of these men was reduced by 1.4 inches after six weeks. Importantly, waist circumference was highly correlated with belly fat, suggesting that just six weeks of interval sprinting training—which called for eighteen twenty-minute sessions, for a total of only six hours of interval sprinting—significantly reduced belly fat.

The Fitness, Muscle Mass, and Insulin-Resistance Response to Aerobic, Resistance, and Interval Sprinting Exercise

Reducing belly fat is a key feature of interval sprinting, but there are other important adaptations that have beneficial implications for health, including increased aerobic fitness and skeletal muscle mass, and a decrease in insulin resistance.

Aerobic Fitness

Aerobic fitness, typically called aerobic power by exercise physiologists, is vital for health. Maximum aerobic fitness is typically measured by getting subjects to exercise to exhaustion on a cycle or treadmill. Gases are collected to assess the ability of an individual to deliver and use oxygen to the exercising muscles. Oxygen, of course, is delivered to the exercising muscles by way of your red blood cells. Researchers at the University of South Carolina found that a lack of aerobic fitness was strongly associated with early mortality.[15] Thus, fitter adults suffered fewer deaths from cancer, heart disease, and stroke. These researchers showed that low aerobic fitness accounted for 16 percent of all deaths in a large group of American adults. This 16 percent contribution to total mortality is significantly higher than other risk factors, such as obesity, smoking, high cholesterol, and diabetes. It has been well documented that being aerobically fit helps reduce the risk for heart disease, metabolic disease, certain cancers, and Alzheimer's disease. The good news is that interval sprinting significantly increases aerobic fitness even though the sprinting exercise is mostly *an*aerobic. We found that fifteen weeks of interval sprinting resulted in a 26 percent increase in the aerobic fitness of young women, compared with a 19 percent increase in another group that completed fifteen weeks of moderate aerobic exercise.[16] The interval sprinting consisted of three twenty-minute sessions per week, compared with three forty-minute sessions of aerobic cycling. In a second study with young, overweight women, we found that twelve weeks of interval sprinting brought an 18 percent increase in aerobic fitness, while young, overweight men saw a 16 percent increase.[17] Thus, a very important characteristic of interval sprinting is that it produces large increases in aerobic fitness. As interval sprinting is mostly anaerobic in nature, it also results in large increases in anaerobic fitness.

Skeletal Muscle Mass

Retaining or increasing skeletal muscle mass is very important when it comes to your health. For example, women with less muscle mass face a higher incidence of the bone-thinning disorder osteoporosis. We typically lose a significant amount of muscle mass as we age, as do people of any age who go on starvation diets. As can be seen in table 4, women who went on a starvation diet, reducing their daily caloric intake by 50 percent, lost about 6.6 pounds of muscle over a sixteen-week period. Since it has been estimated that an increase of 2.2 pounds of skeletal muscle could burn just under 6.6 pounds of fat per year, any loss in muscle mass can result in a reduced incidence of fat loss.

Unfortunately, even exercising diligently does not prevent muscle loss when dieting. When women performed either aerobic or resistance exercise while on a starvation diet, they still lost muscle mass, although the depletion was reduced by between 40 percent and 50 percent. It is well documented that participating in aerobic exercise does not change muscle mass, whereas moderately hard resistance exercise may increase muscle mass for some. As table 4 demonstrates, three interval sprinting studies showed significant increases of leg and trunk muscle mass of 0.7 pounds and 0.9 pounds for women and 1.1 pounds and 1.5 pounds for men, respectively. Our study that examined interval sprinting and dieting is particularly interesting: we asked overweight women to switch to a Mediterranean eating plan, which resulted in their consuming 13 percent fewer calories per day. Despite eating slightly less every day, the women still increased significantly the amount of muscle in their legs (0.7 pounds) and trunk (0.7 pounds) and reduced their body fat by 5.7 pounds after twelve weeks of interval sprinting. These findings suggest that combining a healthy diet, such as the Mediterranean eating plan, with twelve weeks of interval sprinting may be the optimal way to lose belly fat and enhance muscle mass.

Intervention	Weight loss	Fat-free mass loss/gain	Daily caloric decrease
LCD alone	-24.5 pounds	-6.8 pounds	50 percent
LCD with aerobic exercise	-25.1 pounds	-3.3 pounds	50 percent
LCD with resistance exercise	-25.6 pounds	-4.4 pounds	50 percent
ND with interval sprinting (female)	-3.3 pounds	+1.3 pounds	none
MD with interval sprinting	-4.2 pounds	+1.1 pounds	13 percent
ND with interval sprinting (male)	-3.3 pounds	+2.6 pounds	none

Table 4. Comparison of muscle mass loss with no dieting (ND), moderate dieting (MD), and low-calorie dieting (LCD) with or without aerobic, resistance, and interval sprinting exercise

Adapted from information in studies by Kuk, et al., Trapp, et al., Dunn, et al., and Boutcher. [18]

Insulin Resistance

Insulin resistance is measured by assessing the amount of insulin and glucose in the blood. If these levels are high, it indicates that a person's tissues, especially the skeletal muscles and liver, are becoming resistant to the effects of insulin. Insulin, as you may recall, is released from the pancreas when we eat sugar. It enables the sugar in the blood to enter the tissues, to be used as energy by the cells or to be stored as glycogen for later use. Only insulin and exercise can remove sugar from the blood. Failure to reduce blood sugar levels over time is bad for health and typically leads to the development of type 2 diabetes. Participation in all forms of interval sprinting, aerobic exercise, and resistance exercise typically decreases insulin resistance, and we found a large decrease in insulin resistance in two of our studies. The women who participated in the twelve-week study reduced their incidence of insulin resistance by 31 percent, while those in the fifteen-week study experienced a reduction of 36 percent.[16, 17] In our study with overweight young women, their insulin resistance decreased dramatically after six weeks of interval sprinting. In comparison, other studies have found that using aerobic exercise programs lasting longer than twelve weeks typically result in decreased insulin resistance of around 12 percent. Surprisingly, regular resistance exercise also decreases insulin resistance but the exercise has to be moderately hard.

Table 5 was constructed by reviewing the results of articles that examined the maximum oxygen uptake, muscle mass, and insulin-resistance-reduction response to aerobic training, resistance training, and interval training. Although fewer interval sprinting studies have been completed, this form of exercise has brought about equally positive or more positive changes in maximum oxygen uptake, muscle mass, and insulin resistance than both aerobic and resistance exercise.

The typical amount of reduction of insulin resistance in

study participants in randomized, controlled studies lasting greater than two weeks was between 20 percent and 50 percent. We now think that interval sprinting is especially suitable for individuals who suffer from type 2 diabetes and metabolic syndrome.

	Interval sprinting	Aerobic exercise	Resistance exercise
Maximum oxygen uptake increase	16 percent to 25 percent	12 percent to 20 percent	No change
Muscle mass increase	1.1 pounds to 2.6 pounds	No change	1.1 pounds to 2.6 pounds
Insulin-resistance reduction	20 percent to 50 percent	Around 12 percent	Around 10 percent
Average hours of exercise	12–15 hours	36–48 hours	36–48 hours

Table 5. Summary of maximum oxygen uptake, muscle mass, and insulin-resistance-reduction response to aerobic, resistance, and interval training in randomized, controlled trials lasting at least twelve weeks

Interval Sprinting and Special Populations

There are now over fifty articles published in scientific literature examining different aspects of interval training. Surprisingly, a number of these papers have studied the effects of interval training on the health of special populations, including men and women with heart disease, intermittent claudication, diabetes, and depression, as well as on older people, postmenopausal women, and postpregnant women.

Interval training protocols in these studies have varied, but most research groups have used longer interval exercise at less than all-out intensity for two minutes, followed by low-intensity exercise or rest for four minutes. Thus, although cycling for two minutes cannot be classed as sprinting, the exercise was still performed at high intensity and followed by a rest. Although more research needs to be conducted in this area, the preliminary results are promising.

Heart Disease Patients

The heart is the organ that pumps blood to all body tissues; if it stops pumping, death follows quickly. There are a number of heart diseases but two major ones are coronary artery disease and chronic heart disease. Coronary artery disease occurs when the arteries that provide oxygen-bearing blood to the heart become blocked. This lack of oxygenated blood to the heart can damage or destroy the cardiac tissue. Also if a blood clot should form or lodge in the narrowed arteries, preventing blood from reaching the heart, a heart attack, or myocardial infarction, can occur. Blocked arteries in the heart can be caused by smoking, high cholesterol, hypertension, type 2 diabetes, and genetic inheritance. The arteries that supply blood to the heart become narrowed due to a buildup of cholesterol and other material, called plaque, on and inside their inner walls. Chronic heart disease is a condition where the heart does not pump normally and is usually caused by a weak cardiac muscle or faulty heart valves. Heart disease is the major cause of death in most Westernized countries.

A number of studies have investigated the effect of interval training on patients suffering from coronary heart disease and chronic heart failure. A series of studies carried out on coronary-artery bypass surgery patients by one research team in the 1990s showed that, compared with healthy groups of volunteers, their physical performance improved significantly after a program of interval training.[19] Coronary-artery bypass surgery improves blood flow to the heart by grafting a healthy artery or vein from the body to the blocked artery.

Another team examined the effect of interval exercise on stent function following heart surgery. A stent is a small mesh tube that surgeons insert inside a narrow or weak artery to improve blood flow. Results showed that high-intensity interval exercise improved stent function, increased aerobic fitness, and reduced inflammation.[20] A different study compared the effects of aerobic interval training and moderate continuous aerobic training on aerobic fitness and quality of life after a coronary-artery bypass graft.[21] Four weeks of interval and continuous aerobic exercise showed a significant increase in aerobic fitness of all participants; however, six months later, the interval group had greater aerobic fitness than the continuous exercise group. Interval training protocols in these studies involved cycling at less than all-out intensity for two minutes, immediately followed by rest for four minutes.

With regard to chronic heart disease patients, one study found that sixteen weeks of high-intensity interval training enhanced their functional capacity and quality of life.[22] Another compared the effect of moderate aerobic and high-intensity exercise on cardiovascular function in heart failure patients. Heart failure is a condition caused by the heart not efficiently pumping blood around the body. Aerobic fitness was increased more with aerobic interval training and was associated with greater improvements in the left ventricle, the chamber of the heart responsible for propelling freshly oxygenated blood out to the rest of the body via the large artery known as the aorta.[23] A different study also showed that high-intensity interval exercise was better than moderate continuous aerobic exercise for increasing aerobic fitness in coronary artery patients.[24] Collectively, research examining interval exercise and coronary artery disease and chronic heart failure has found that interval training increases aerobic fitness in far less time than conventional moderate aerobic exercise does. Quality of life was also consistently improved, as were a number of indicators of heart function.[25]

Chronic Obstructive Pulmonary Disease Patients

Chronic obstructive pulmonary disease affects breathing and is characterized by unremitting bronchitis or emphysema, which narrows the airways in the lungs. COPD is typically caused by smoking, which inflames the lungs. In the United States, it is the third leading cause of death and it has been calculated to cost over $42 billion in increased health care and lost productivity. Estimates suggest that chronic obstructive pulmonary disease will become the fourth leading killer worldwide by 2030.

Patients with this disease usually have trouble performing

aerobic exercise and typically have an overall poor quality of life. When performing continuous aerobic exercise, COPD patients typically experience breathing discomfort and have to stop for a rest. As exercising and resting are the basis of interval training, it appears that this form of exercise is suitable for chronic obstructive pulmonary disease patients. A twelve-week study compared interval exercise with aerobic exercise and found that patients with COPD improved their exercise tolerance significantly.[26] Continuous aerobic exercise also improved exercise tolerance but involved twice as much exercise time. After both interval and aerobic exercise, quality of life improved dramatically. These results have been replicated in a number of other studies. In one clinical trial, researchers showed that both interval exercise and continuous moderate aerobic exercise improved muscle function; however, interval training caused fewer problems, such as shortness of breath and breathing discomfort.[27] Interval training protocols in these studies typically entailed less than all-out intensity cycling for thirty seconds, immediately followed by thirty seconds of rest.

Overall, research examining interval exercise and chronic obstructive pulmonary disease has shown that interval sprinting increases aerobic fitness in less time than moderate aerobic exercise does. Quality of life also consistently improved, and, importantly, there were less problems with interval sprint training. Because interval training allows COPD patients to tolerate harder-intensity exercise for longer periods of time with less breathing and leg discomfort, it appears to be superior to other training methods.[28]

Metabolic Syndrome and Diabetic Patients

Metabolic syndrome is a condition distinguished by having a lot of belly fat, high blood pressure, insulin resistance, and poor blood lipid profiles. It is a precursor to type 2 diabetes and is typically an outcome of an unhealthy diet and being sedentary. Type 2 diabetic people have too much sugar in their blood because their bodies become resistant to the hormone insulin. Type 2 diabetes can be prevented but not cured. The incidence of type 2 diabetes has increased substantially during the past fifty years along with rates of obesity: in 2010 there were about 285 million people diagnosed with metabolic syndrome compared with about 30 million in 1985. Long-term complications caused by type 2 diabetes are heart disease, stroke, retinopathy (damage to the retina of the eye), kidney disease, and nerve degeneration. In contrast to type 2 diabetes, type 1 diabetes results from the inability of the pancreas to produce insulin. The degradation of the organ's beta cells is usually brought about by the immune system. In Western countries, type 1 diabetes makes up about 10 percent of the total diabetic population. Most people who develop type 1 diabetes are usually of average weight and healthy in comparison with those who develop type 2 diabetes. Type 1 diabetics are dependent on taking insulin in addition to observing certain dietary measures, whereas people with type 2 can usually manage the disease through diet and anti-diabetic medications. Fortunately, most type 2 diabetics do not have to inject insulin although eventually many of them *will* require it.

Aerobic exercise has been shown to be beneficial for

reducing symptoms of metabolic syndrome and type 2 diabetes. The effects of interval training, however, have been examined less, but initial results are promising. For instance, one study placed thirty-two metabolic syndrome patients on a sixteen-week interval training program and found that many health risk factors were reversed.[29] Another looked at the effects of resistance and interval exercise training on skeletal muscle function in people with type 2 diabetes.[30] They found that ten weeks of resistance and interval training in unfit type 2 diabetic patients brought improvements in muscle function and blood pressure. Interval training protocols in these studies consisted of moderately strenuous cycling for two minutes, followed immediately by four minutes of rest. In a subsequent clinical trial, low-volume interval sprinting—ten sixty-second bouts of cycling with each bout followed by a sixty-second rest period for twenty minutes—rapidly improved the volunteers' glucose control and induced beneficial skeletal muscle adaptations.[31]

The effects of a single ten-second sprint on exercising type 1 diabetics' glucose levels have also been investigated. It is well established that moderate-intensity aerobic exercise increases the risk of hypoglycemia (low blood sugar levels) following physical exertion in those with type 1 diabetes. This study found that adding a ten-second maximum sprint at the end of moderate aerobic exercise prevented a drop in blood sugar levels.[32] In yet another study of glucose levels following exercise, researchers reported that levels remained more stable in the subjects who took part in thirty minutes of interval sprinting than in those who performed thirty minutes of continuous aerobic exercise.[33]

Collectively, research examining interval exercise and metabolic diseases such as type 2 diabetes has shown that interval training consistently increases insulin sensitivity and reverses a number of risk factors.[34]

Depressed Individuals

Depression is a long-term mood disorder and is usually defined as having continuous unhappiness and reduced enjoyment of everyday life for more than two weeks. It has been estimated that about one in seven people in Westernized countries are clinically depressed. People who experience depression typically have a range of health problems, such as cardiovascular disease, headaches, back pain, anxiety attacks, and poor-quality sleep. Depressed individuals exhibit chronically elevated cortisol levels, which stimulates belly fat accumulation.

In 2008, investigators from Amsterdam found that depressed people had twice the risk of gaining belly fat over a five-year period compared with people without depression. These authors suggested that storing fat in the belly puts depressed people at much greater risk for cardiovascular disease and diabetes.

Interestingly, the investigators reported no association between depression and obesity. This finding suggests that, despite being of normal weight, depressed people had elevated levels of belly fat. Another study, this one of middle-aged African American and Caucasian women, drew a similar conclusion. The researchers found a strong relationship between depression and belly fat but no association between depression levels and subcutaneous fat. Although it is not clear how depression causes an increase in belly fat, one mechanism might be that it increases the production of cortisol and inflammatory compounds.

Research has shown that all kinds of moderately vigorous exercise tend to alleviate clinical depression. For depression reduction, moderately vigorous exercise such as fast walking, jogging, and strength training produced better results than easy exercise did. Depression has been shown to subside in weeks; however, longer exercise programs seem to produce greater reductions in depression levels. Whether or not the positive effect of exercise on depression is related to decreased belly fat is unknown. That longer, moderately vigorous exercise tends to alleviate clinical depression more may indicate that these kinds of exercise programs result in a greater reduction of belly fat.

The effect of interval sprinting on depression has not been examined in formal studies. However, given the large reductions in belly fat occurring after interval sprinting and the connection between belly fat and depression, its potential appears to be significant. Interval sprinting may be suitable for depressed patients because it can be fun, can be performed in a group, is time efficient, and has been shown to reduce belly fat.

Intermittent Claudication Patients

Intermittent claudication is skeletal muscle pain experienced as aching, cramping, and numbness, which usually occurs in the calf muscles when walking and is relieved only by resting. Intermittent claudication is due to peripheral artery disease brought about by blockages of the arteries of the leg. People who smoke, have high blood pressure, or possess type 2 diabetes have a greater incidence of intermittent claudication. Men over fifty have the highest incidence, and it affects around 5 percent of people in Western populations.

A number of studies have shown that regular aerobic exercise can improve intermittent claudication symptoms. Patients typically walk for five minutes, rest for five minutes, and then repeat this pattern for twenty to thirty minutes. However, one study found that high-intensity training at 80 percent of maximum oxygen uptake was more effective than an identical volume of low-intensity training for improving aerobic fitness in patients with intermittent claudication.[35] Maximal oxygen uptake is the maximal rate at which oxygen can be used by the body during exhaustive exercise. It is a measure of aerobic fitness and is usually assessed by exercising an individual to exhaustion on a stationary cycle or treadmill. The high-intensity training patients carried out two minutes of speed walking on a treadmill, followed by three-minute sit-down resting periods. This was performed eight times. Another study conducted a high-intensity rehabilitation program with intermittent claudication patients that lasted twelve weeks. Patients walked on a treadmill for six minutes at a speed that brought about ischemia and maximum claudication pain. Ischemia is a medical term describing what happens when the heart doesn't get enough oxygen. When patients reached this level, they stopped walking and rested for three minutes. Patients performed this protocol six times per session. Results showed that those patients who successfully completed the six sessions showed the greatest decrease in claudication symptoms. The authors concluded that, as no adverse events were experienced, patients with intermittent claudication can safely tolerate high-intensity exercise programs.[36]

Obese and Overweight Adults and Children

Obesity is a condition in which body and belly fat accumulation negatively affects health. It increases an individual's chances of heart disease, type 2 diabetes, sleep apnea, and certain cancer types. Obese individuals also have a reduced life expectancy. People are classified as obese when their BMI is 30 or greater. Obesity is typically caused by genetic influences, eating to excess, and being sedentary, although some people can become obese because of endocrine disorders and certain medications. There has been a dramatic increase in overweight and obesity over the past fifty years in both developed and developing countries.

For obese and overweight individuals, regular aerobic exercise has only a minor effect on total body fat, unless they are prepared to exercise for at least one hour, five times per week. The good news is that just one hour a week of interval sprinting significantly reduces total body fat in these men and women who possessed an average BMI of 28.[37] Other researchers studied the effects of a twelve-week, high-intensity exercise program on obese older men and women and found a significant reduction in belly fat, while subjects in a moderate-intensity group showed no decrease.[38] Similarly, another study found that interval training significantly reduced belly fat in older men and women.[39] Importantly, they discovered that reductions in belly fat were strongly related to reductions in insulin resistance: the greater the reduction in belly fat, the greater the improvement in insulin sensitivity.

With regard to childhood obesity, one study compared the effects of high-intensity exercise and a multitreatment strategy on a number of cardiovascular risk factors in obese adolescents.[40] One group performed aerobic interval training twice per week for twelve weeks: four minutes of hard uphill running on a treadmill, followed by four minutes of rest. Another group undertook a multidisciplinary approach over twelve months, including dietary changes, moderate exercise, and psychological counseling twice a month. The results? The youngsters who engaged in high-intensity exercise saw a greater reduction in their cardiovascular risk factors than the multitreatment group did.

Overall, research examining the effects of high-intensity exercise and interval sprinting exercise on the obese and overweight has shown that this kind of exercise decreases body fat to a greater extent than continuous aerobic exercise. Belly fat has been shown to be reduced by interval sprint training in far less time than by aerobic exercise. Because interval training, especially on the stationary bike, is easily performed by obese adults and children, and because it results in more subcutaneous and belly fat loss, it appears to be superior to other kinds of training.[41]

Postmenopausal Women

Premenopausal women are typically younger than forty-six and tend to have less belly fat than men, as they store their fat in their legs, hips, and on the backs of their arms. This differing pattern of fat storage for women and men is mainly an outcome of the hormone estrogen. As women go through menopause in their late forties and early fifties, however, estrogen production stops or slows down, resulting in increased belly fat accumulation. Scientists have suggested that the estrogen reduction is accompanied by an increase in the stress hormone cortisol, which, as mentioned previously, helps increase belly fat. Thus, women older than forty-six tend to have greater increases in belly fat than males do. Women in their late forties can find their waistlines increasing even if they don't gain much weight, as increasing belly fat forces the abdominal wall outward.

Importantly, diet is relatively ineffective at reducing the belly fat stores of postmenopausal women. In one study, postmenopausal women lost belly fat only when exercise, in the form of walking, was added to a diet. Interval training, however, has been shown to result in greater belly fat reductions in postmenopausal women. The aforementioned study of middle-aged men and women showed a 48 percent decrease in belly fat, measured by MRI, with an 18 percent decrease in subcutaneous fat after steady-state aerobic exercise two days per week and interval training one day a week for eight weeks.[42] Another study, of thirty-two middle-aged men and women with metabolic syndrome, entailed interval training three times per week for sixteen weeks. The participants' aerobic fitness was enhanced by 26 percent, whereas their body weight decreased by 5.1 pounds.[43]

Overall, research examining the effect of interval exercise on postmenopausal women's health has shown that interval training or sprinting increases aerobic fitness in less time than moderate aerobic exercise does. Body fat also decreases to a greater extent after interval training interventions compared with continuous aerobic exercise. Interval training has also been shown to reduce belly fat in far less time than aerobic exercise does.

Pregnancy and Interval Sprinting

Many women increase their food intake excessively when pregnant, and while there are general guidelines to help women understand how much weight gain is appropriate during pregnancy, there are no specific recommendations regarding the amount of fat they should include. Weight gain during pregnancy is influenced by the baby's weight and the mother's increase in blood volume and body fat. Some fat stores are increased during pregnancy to enhance breastfeeding, but excessive fat gain increases a number of health risks for mother and baby. Unfortunately, a significant number of women increase their belly fat stores during pregnancy. Although many women think they have to "eat for two" when pregnant, only a small amount of extra calories are needed. While pregnant women should not be encouraged to diet to lose weight, as this may harm the health of the growing baby, a healthy diet and regular physical activity are important for the long-term health of both mother and baby.

But what about after pregnancy? Given that many women will retain their increased belly fat stores after giving birth, and that interval sprinting has been shown to decrease belly fat in nonpregnant women, it follows that interval sprinting may be the optimal exercise for reducing these unwanted belly fat stores. Research studies, however, are needed to confirm this relationship.

With regard to conception, no studies have investigated the effect of interval training on conception rates. Some research has been done with aerobic exercise, and it seems that really hard exercise, like marathon training, is detrimental, while moderate exercise—three forty-five-minute sessions of aerobic exercise per week, for example—is beneficial for conception. So where would interval sprinting fit in? Interval sprinting is performed at a harder intensity but is much shorter than a forty-five-minute bout of aerobic exercise. In our studies with women ages eighteen to thirty, we did not have any reports of menstrual irregularity after training three times per week for twelve or fifteen weeks. With regard to belly fat and conception, it has been shown that those women possessing elevated belly fat stores have a reduced rate of conception. As interval sprinting has been shown to reduce belly fat in women, it is feasible that interval sprinting may enhance conception rates, but research into this area is required.

*

In the research described above, all subjects or patients were screened medically before participating in high-intensity interval training. It is important that you seek medical advice on the possible positive or negative effects of interval training on your health before beginning an interval sprinting regime. The potential interaction between any medication you might be taking and interval training should also be estimated. For example, if you have heart disease and are taking some form of beta-blocker, you will not be able to elevate your heart rate to the recommended level during exercise.

The ideal team to help as you embark on an interval training program consists of a physician who is supportive of lifestyle-change strategies and a Registered Clinical Exercise Physiologist (RCEP) qualified to advise you on exercise as well as diet, stress management, and sleep-quality enhancement. Together they will be able to guide you on what form of exercise is right for you, how long each session should last, how many times per week you should exercise, and at what intensity. You can find more information on RCEPs by visiting http://certification.acsm.org.

If you are interested just in improving your fitness and health, then most types of continuous, steady-state exercise will be effective. However, if you want to lose belly fat and improve your insulin sensitivity—as well as improve your aerobic and anaerobic fitness and increase muscle mass— then interval sprinting is the best option. See chapter 3 for more information on incorporating the interval sprinting program into your life.

*

This chapter has outlined the way we should exercise if we want to lose belly fat. It's important to remember the following:

- Aerobic exercise can bring about a decrease in belly fat but demands exercising at a moderately hard intensity for at least five hours per week.

- Resistance exercise does not seem to decrease belly fat in most people.

- Interval sprinting has resulted in a 17 percent decrease in belly fat when males exercised for one hour per week for twelve weeks.

- We're not sure how interval exercise works on belly fat, but it's likely that increased fat burning during and after exercise and possibly appetite suppression are the main factors.

- Interval training has been used successfully in a number of special populations, such as heart disease patients and people with type 2 diabetes.

Chapter 3
The Interval Sprinting Belly Fat Loss Program

Now that you're familiar with how belly fat affects your health and the positive effects that interval sprinting can have on the amount of belly fat you carry, let's outline an eight-second-sprint/twelve-second-recovery interval sprinting program. This chapter will also explain the benefits such a program offers, the equipment you'll need, and how to begin training.

What Happens to Heart Rate and Hormones During Interval Sprinting?

Heart Rate

Your body undergoes a number of acute responses to interval sprinting, but the three most essential for losing belly fat involve heart rate, the blood's levels of lactate, and fat-burning hormones. Your heart-rate response depends on what type of interval sprinting protocol you undertake, but typically it is significantly elevated during interval sprinting exercise and declines slightly during the recovery between sprints. For example, peak heart rates during the hard Wingate test typically exceed 170 beats per minute during an all-out cycle sprint of thirty seconds, with the average heart rate across the thirty-second sprint being 150 beats per minute. Studies have found a smaller heart-rate response for an interval sprinting protocol consisting of ten six-second sprints interspersed with a thirty-second recovery.[1] Heart rate increased to 142 beats per minute after the first sprint and then increased to 173 beats per minute following the tenth sprint.[2] As can be seen in figure 5, the heart rates of young adults gradually increase during the twenty minutes of eight-second/twelve-second interval sprinting. In the eight-second/twelve-second program, there is typically a small heart-rate decrease of around 3 to 5 beats per minute during each recovery period.

Heart-rate response to interval sprinting varies depending on your age. In young adults, heart rate typically averages around 150 beats per minute after five minutes of interval sprinting, which then increases to 160 beats per minute after twenty minutes of exercise. For middle-aged adults, optimal heart-rate response is generally lower: around 140 beats per minute after five minutes of interval sprinting and increasing to 150 beats per minute after twenty minutes of exercise.

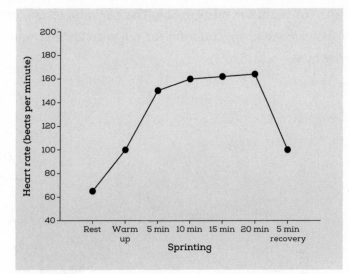

Figure 5. The heart-rate response of young adults to one session of interval sprinting consisting of an eight-second sprint and twelve seconds of easy pedalling for twenty minutes.

Measuring Heart Rate

Heart rate during exercise and recovery can be measured manually or by a heart-rate monitor. The best place to measure heart rate during exercise or exercise recovery using the manual method is at the radial artery, located in the wrist. The fingers should be used to locate a pulse rather than the thumb.

To locate the radial pulse on your wrist, position the index and middle fingers on the opposite wrist, approximately a half inch on the inside of the wrist, below the index finger. (See figure 6.) When you feel your pulse, count the number of beats for one minute. The per-minute rate can also be calculated by counting for ten seconds and multiplying by 6.

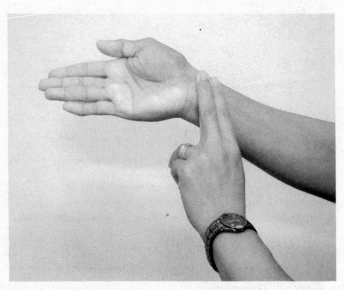

Figure 6. Locating the radial pulse at the base of the wrist.

A heart-rate monitor is much easier and gives a much more accurate reading of your heart rate than doing it manually. There are numerous heart-rate smartphone apps available for iPhones and Android devices that can measure heart rate. Using a heart-rate monitor, as pictured in figure 7, is also useful when you want to record your heart rates in order to review them later. Such monitors also allow you to download your records to a computer.

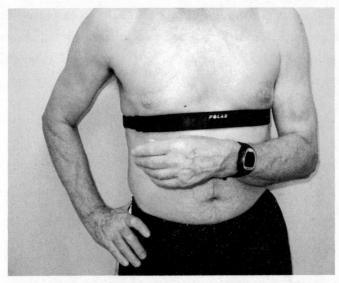

Figure 7. Assessing heart rate by using a heart-rate monitor.

Rating of Perceived Exertion (RPE)

Exercise physiologists use a system called "rating of perceived exertion scale" to measure how hard people feel they are exerting themselves during exercise. (See appendix D, page 189.) While exercising, people are asked to express their perceived effort level on a scale of 6 to 20.[3] When performing lower-intensity interval sprinting such as the eight-second-sprint/twelve-second-recovery program, the rating of perceived exertion is usually around 12 and increases to just over 15 by the end of the session. This can be seen in figure 8 (following).

When performing aerobic exercise, the rating is typically equivalent to about one-tenth of the exercise heart rate. Thus, a rating of 16 would typically accompany a heart rate of 160 beats per minute for young adults in their twenties. For aerobic exercise, if you increase the intensity of exercise as you get fitter, your rating of perceived exertion typically stays the same.

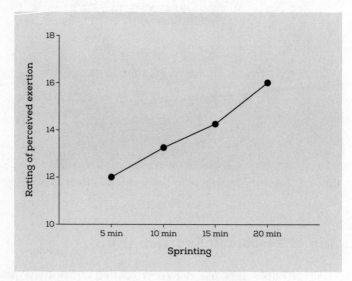

Figure 8. The RPE response of young adults to one session of interval sprinting consisting of an eight-second sprint and twelve seconds of easy pedalling for twenty minutes.

But with interval sprinting exercise, the rating is generally equivalent to about one-eleventh of the exercising heart rate, so a rating of 14 would typically accompany a heart rate of 150 beats per minute for young adults. As people get fitter with repeated interval sprinting, they increase pedal rate and resistance. After interval training, however, instead of staying the same, the RPE tends to go up.[4] This is probably because the greater force developed by skeletal muscles needed to cope with higher pedal-resistance loads causes higher exertional perceptions. Thus, as force production increases, the greater amount of signalling received by the brain's sensory centers could be why the rating of perceived exertion climbs after interval sprinting training.

Blood Lactate Level

The chemical lactate builds up in the blood when you take on anaerobic exercise, which is performed at a higher intensity than aerobic exercise. Anaerobic exercise uses energy systems that do not require oxygen—relying mainly on glycolysis to release energy into the muscles—and is typically brought into action when you perform brief, high-intensity bouts of exercise continuously, as with interval sprinting. Glycolysis is the metabolic pathway that converts glucose into pyruvate, which produces a high-energy compound called ATP. Heavy use of glycolysis during this kind of exercise results in enhanced acidity in the exercising muscles—lactate—which then spills into the circulation.

Exercise physiologists measure blood lactate levels to gauge how much energy is being derived from the glycolytic pathways. Blood lactate levels are low while you're at rest but can increase significantly during anaerobic exercise. For example, blood lactate levels during the high-intensity Wingate test are typically six to ten times higher than those at rest. Lactate levels gradually increase during longer, lower-intensity interval sprinting protocols such as the eight-second/twelve-second sprint for twenty minutes, and they are usually between two and four times greater than those at rest after five minutes of interval sprinting for both trained cyclists and untrained women who took part in our study. (See figure 9.) Lactate levels were about five times greater than those at rest after fifteen minutes of interval sprinting. Thus, lactate levels immediately increase at the start of interval sprinting and continue to increase slowly throughout the exercise session. Despite increasing lactate levels during sprinting exercise, it appears that fat transport is also increased. For example, a twenty-minute session of eight-second/twelve-second sprinting resulted in elevated levels of free fatty acids in the blood.[5]

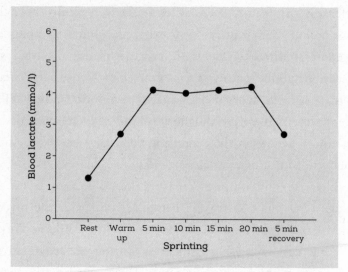

Figure 9. Blood lactate response of young adults to one session of interval sprinting consisting of an eight-second sprint and twelve seconds of easy pedalling for twenty minutes.

Blood lactate levels gradually increase during interval sprinting such as the eight-second/twelve-second sprint for twenty minutes protocol and are usually three to four times greater than resting values at the end of a twenty-minute session.

Hormones

Hormones that have been found to increase during interval sprinting include catecholamines and growth hormone, both of which are integral to fat release and burning. Catecholamine response is typically elevated after Wingate sprints for both men and women, while the response to less-intensive interval sprinting has also been shown to be higher. For example, norepinephrine response to long-bout (twenty-four-second sprint/thirty-six-second recovery) and short-bout (six-second sprint/nine-second recovery) intermittent treadmill exercise was significantly elevated postexercise. Our study also found significantly elevated epinephrine and norepinephrine levels after twenty minutes of interval sprinting cycle exercise—eight-second/twelve-second and twenty-four-second/thirty-six-second programs—in trained and untrained young women. (See figure 10, page 78.)[6] Catecholamines are hormones made by the adrenal glands. The main catecholamines are norepinephrine and epinephrine, which when released into the blood cause fat cells to release their fatty acids. Another study examined the catecholamine response of twelve males who performed ten six-second cycle sprints with a thirty-second recovery between sprints. Compared with baseline, the level of epinephrine in the blood increased 6.3 times, whereas norepinephrine increased 14.5 times at the end of sprinting.[7] This large catecholamine response to interval sprinting is in contrast to moderate, steady-state aerobic exercise, which typically brings about small increases in epinephrine and norepinephrine. The interval sprinting catecholamine response is an important finding, as catecholamines are the major drivers of fat release from both belly and muscle depots.

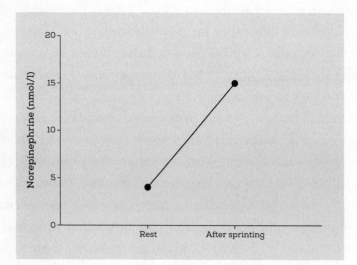

Figure 10. The norepinephrine response of young adults to one session of interval sprinting consisting of an eight-second sprint and twelve seconds of easy pedalling for twenty minutes.

Growth hormone, which also induces fat burning by coaxing fat cells to release fat, has been found to increase during high-intensity exercise. With regard to interval sprinting, one study investigated the growth-hormone response to thirty-second treadmill sprinting.[8] Male and female athletes displayed a marked growth-hormone response, and there was a greater growth-hormone response for sprint exercise compared with endurance training. This suggests that regular interval sprint training increases growth-hormone levels. In this study, the hormone concentration was still ten times higher than baseline levels after sixty minutes of recovery.

How to Perform Interval Cycle Sprinting

The eight-second-sprint/twelve-second-recovery pedalling cadence is recommended. It is best to wear shorts, but a track-suit bottom can be worn, as long as it does not get caught in the pedals. Trainers are suitable for footwear, and when cycling inside, it is a good idea to have a towel handy to wipe off excess sweat. In average temperature conditions (68°F to 75°F), you'll typically lose around 0.7 pounds of sweat after twenty minutes of interval sprinting. You can measure your sweat loss during exercise simply by measuring your nude weight before and immediately after an interval sprinting session: if you weigh 154.3 pounds nude before sprinting and 153.6 pounds nude after the session, then you would have lost 0.7 pounds of perspiration. Sweat loss is usually significantly greater when exercising in hot, humid conditions.

Choosing a Stationary Bike

First, choose a bike of sufficient quality to withstand sprint-ing at high pedal rates. Of the range of stationary bikes available, the most suitable ones for interval sprinting allow you to set a pedal resistance that is independent of power output. Some of the newer electronic bikes do not allow you to do this, so when you sprint against a pedal resistance of 2.2 pounds, for example, instead of the resistance staying the same in the recovery phase, the bike will increase the resistance to produce the same amount of work generated during the sprinting phase. What should be easy pedalling during the recovery phase becomes hard exercise, and having a strenuous recovery phase will prevent the body from removing the waste products produced during sprinting. It will also make the workout excessively demanding, tiring you out more quickly.

HOW TO SET UP THE BIKE

Adjust the saddle height so that when you're sitting on the bike, you have about a 5 percent bend at the knee. Then raise or lower the handlebars so that your hands rest on top of them. Make sure that the pedals have foot grips. The correct setup for sprinting is shown in figure 11.

CHOOSING THE PEDAL RATE AND RESISTANCE

We know that the catecholamine production during bike interval sprinting is brought about by moving the legs quickly: cycling fast is more important than cycling hard. Your pedal rate will be influenced by a range of factors, such as your fitness, age, health, leg muscle mass, and height. It is best to start with a comfortable pedal rate and then increase it if your rating of perceived exertion is less than 12 and your heart rate is low for your age.

The pedal rate is more important than the load. This

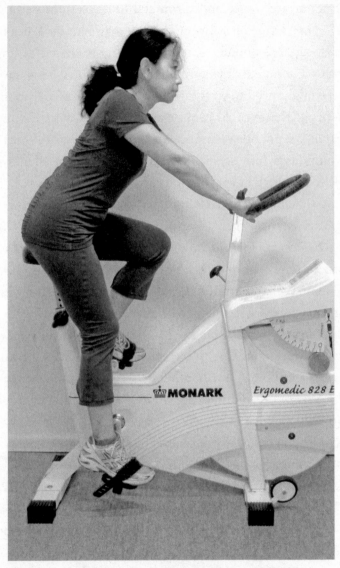

Figure 11. The setup for performing interval sprinting on a stationary bike.

means that a woman with no health issues could start on a 1.1-pound resistance and sprint at 100 revolutions per minute (rpm). Fitter or stronger women may require a heavier load—say, 2.2 pounds—and sprint at more than 100 revolutions a minute, while a smaller, older female who is out of shape might need to start at a pedal resistance of 1.1 pounds and a pedal rate of 90 rpm. A perfectly healthy man should start at 2.2 pounds resistance and a pedal rate of 100 to 110 revolutions a minute, while fitter, stronger men should be able to sprint at 115 revolutions a minute or greater.

Stationary bikes have a number of different ways to vary pedal resistance. Increasing pedal resistance is like cycling up a hill: the steeper the hill, the greater the pedal resistance. Stationary bikes typically control pedal resistance by either tightening a band around the wheel or by slowing the wheel with magnets. Most bikes will quantify pedal resistance in kilograms or pounds. On the Monark bike made in Sweden, for example, tightening the strap on the wheel from 0.5 kilograms (1.1 pounds) to 1.0 kilograms (2.2 pounds) when pedalling at 100 revolutions per minute will double the power output, which is how much power you are generating when cycling and is typically measured in watts. To calculate your power, or watts, simply multiply the pedal rate by the pedal resistance. Thus, cycling at 100 rpm at a resistance of 2.2 pounds is equivalent to a power output of 100 watts. If all this sounds too technical, don't worry. Most people, in their first session, should try to pedal at a rate of 100 revolutions per minute with a resistance of 1.1 pounds.

You will have to increase the load and pedal rate as your fitness improves. For the first week of training, if you're not in shape, try ten minutes of interval sprinting and then see how you feel at the end of the session and when you wake up the next morning. If everything is fine, increase the exercise time to fifteen minutes during week two. By week three, most people should be able to complete the full twenty minutes of interval sprinting.

After two to three weeks, you will probably find that your sprint pedal rate is too low. If your rating of perceived exertion is 12 or less, increase the pedal rate by 5 rpm—for example, from 90 to 95—and see how your RPE and heart rate change.

Heart Rate and Rating of Perceived Exertion During Interval Sprinting

Monitoring your heart rate is important, although working out your optimal interval sprinting heart rate is tricky. Typically, to determine exercise heart rate, exercise physiologists calculate an individual's maximum exercise heart rate by continually increasing the power output on a bike until the person reaches exhaustion and his or her heart rate will not increase any further. Maximum heart rates typically, but not always, lower with age. For instance, a person in his twenties might have a maximum heart rate of 200 beats per minute, whereas a sixty-year-old's might reach 160 beats per minute. For interval sprinting, the optimal heart rate is typically around 75 percent to 80 percent of a person's true maximum heart rate: for a young person, an exercise heart rate averaging 150 beats per minute would be appropriate, while for a seventy-year-old, an average of 113 beats per minute might be optimal.

Unfortunately, most people do not know their maximum heart rate. It can be estimated by using something called the Karvonen formula, which simply calculates the required heart rate by subtracting the person's age from 220. Thus, a twenty-year-old would have an estimated maximum heart rate of 200 beats per minute (220 minus 20 equals 200). For someone aged sixty: 160 beats per minute (220 minus 60 equals 160). However, young people can have a maximum heart rate of 160 beats per minute and older people, especially if they are fit, of over 200 beats per minute.

If you do not know your true maximum heart rate, the best approach is trial and error. For example, an unfit but healthy twenty-year-old male could start interval sprinting using a pedal rate of 100 revolutions per minute at a resistance of 1.1 pounds. If his true maximum heart rate was 200 beats per minute, then his exercise heart rate should be around 150 beats per minute. As discussed below, the rating of perceived exertion for a heart rate of 150 when interval sprinting is around 14—somewhat hard to hard. If the RPE is 17—very hard—then this person's true maximum heart rate is probably lower than 200 beats per minute; therefore, a heart rate of 150 beats per minute when exercising would likely be too much. Optimal target heart rates are around 150 to 160 beats per minute for most people in their twenties, 140 to 150 beats per minute for most people in their thirties, 130 to 140 beats per minute for most people in their forties, 120 to 130 beats per minute for most people in their fifties, and 110 to 120 beats per minute for most people in their sixties.

Heart rate will continue to increase during a twenty-minute session of interval sprinting. Thus, at the start of exercising, you do not want your heart rate to be too high—for example, 160 beats per minute, as it will end up around 170 beats per minute. Heart rate is also affected by heat, which means that exercising in warm, humid conditions will result in much higher heart rates, as the heart has to work harder to cool you by shunting blood to your skin.

It is also important to measure your heart rate at the end of the four-minute cool-down period. If your heart rate got up to 160 beats per minute, it should get down below 100 beats per minute by the end of the cool-down. As you get fitter, your cool-down heart rate should decrease more quickly.

Your First Session of Interval Sprinting

Before starting a high-intensity interval training program, you should be medically screened by a physician or a registered clinical exercise physiologist. This is especially important if you are older, have any risk factors (e.g., obesity, smoking, sedentary lifestyle), have any diseases (e.g., heart disease, hypertension), or are on prescription or OTC medication.

Make sure that you have decided on a suitable pedal rate (90 to 130 rpm for most untrained people) and pedal resistance (between 1.1 pounds and 3.3 pounds). Perform a four-minute warm-up using continuous cycling at 60 to 90 rpm with a resistance of 1.1 pounds. This should yield a rating of perceived exertion of around 11. If your RPE is higher—say, 13—decrease the resistance and pedal rate. Interval sprinting to music makes it much more enjoyable, and while it certainly can be performed without a soundtrack, attempting to time each sprint and recovery session tends to make the experience tedious. Music specifically developed for interval sprinting, called *LifeSprints*, is available on iTunes (see page 199). If you are not using *LifeSprints* music, you need to time the warm-up, sprinting, recovery, and cool-down phases. You can download apps for iPhones and Android devices that allow you to create your own interval sprinting program. The *LifeSprints* music will prompt you to get ready for the sprint through a 3, 2, 1 countdown, and the sprint component of the music is fast, whereas the recovery is slow. Therefore, you have to learn to sprint during the eight-second fast music and slow your pedalling rate during the twelve seconds of slow music. If you are timing yourself, increase your pedal rate three seconds before the actual sprint.

When sprinting, the pedal rate displayed on your bike will always lag behind the real pedal rate, although some bikes do not display or record pedal rate. By the end of the eight-second sprint, the bike should have caught up and be displaying the real pedal rate. It's important that you sense the feeling of your targeted pedal rate so that you can remain consistent throughout the eight-second sprint, without relying on the bike to tell you what your rate is.

When sprinting, it is very important to push and pull with your legs. When you push down on the pedal, you activate the quadriceps muscle, located in the front of your upper thigh, and when you pull up the pedal, you activate the hamstring muscles in the back of your thigh. It is much easier to cycle at high pedal rates if you use this push-pull technique.

If you use only a push action, which is typical for beginners, it makes the sprinting feel much harder. The push-pull technique involves more leg muscle mass and should produce more fat burning. It is advisable to push back slightly on the handlebars with your arms to stabilize your pelvis to prevent rocking and bouncing. This avoids possible soreness after interval sprinting exercise.

What Does Interval Sprinting Feel Like?

For most people, the first couple of sprints of a session feel quite hard, but once they have established a rhythm, it gets easier. Most people will not start breathing heavily until after about five minutes of sprinting; this is also the time they typically start sweating. We think this is because this form of exercise starts to deplete the short-term energy supplies in the exercising muscles after about five minutes, meaning that the body has to switch to sugar stores inside the muscle to provide the fuel for sprinting. Toward the end of the session, fat stored inside the muscle is also used, and it continues to be used during the recovery period. Breathing is likely to become heavier.

As fat burning is more likely to occur in the latter stages of the session, you should keep working at the correct intensity throughout the full twenty minutes. Toward the end, your legs should feel slightly tired. However, you should feel energized rather than exhausted.

It is important to perform the four-minute cool-down so that your heart rate can return to normal before you get off the bike. A pedal rate and resistance lower than your warm-up—for example, 50 revolutions per minute at 1.1 pounds—should see your heart rate go below 100 beats per minute by the end of the cool-down. If your heart rate does not decrease quickly, change your maximum pedal rate and resistance to 50 rpm at 0.6 pounds. Jumping off the bike immediately after sprinting is unadvisable, as it may cause blood to pool in the legs and fainting.

What Is the Best Time of Day to Do Interval Sprinting?

The best time of day for interval sprinting is early in the morning, before breakfast. If you can do it without eating, we believe it will result in increased fat burning. If you can exercise only at lunchtime, try not to eat two to three hours beforehand and drink only water or green tea for as long as possible prior to your session. Exercising at night is probably the second-best option, as long as you can sit down to your evening meal at least two hours before interval sprinting. For example, eating dinner at six o'clock and exercising at 8 o'clock will give time for the insulin in your blood to get taken up by the body's tissues.

As for your postworkout routine, remember that eating sugar and protein elevates the concentration of insulin in your blood and encourages fat storage rather than fat burning, so try to drink only water or green tea for as long as possible. The advantage of exercising at night is that you can avoid eating for at least eight hours afterward because you are asleep, which will allow your body to burn more fat.

Methods of Interval Sprinting

SPRINT CYCLING

Cycling on a stationary bike is probably the optimal form of interval sprinting, as it is non-weight-bearing and thus less stressful on ankles, knees, and hips. Most research examining the effects of interval sprinting has used the stationary bike, and it boasts a number of unique aspects that other forms of exercise do not. For instance, the bike allows people to complete a significant amount of sprinting without feeling exhausted. If a woman uses the eight-second/twelve-second protocol and cycles at a pedal rate of 125 revolutions per minute during sprinting, she would have sprinted 3.7 miles during the twenty minutes of exercise. If her rate was 85 rpm during each rest period, she would have pedalled an additional 3.8 miles, for a total cycling distance of 7.5 miles. The eight-second-sprint protocol involves sixty sprints, resulting in a total of 1,006 pedal revolutions for eight minutes of sprinting during the twenty-minute session. Thus, the optimal interval sprinting protocol would be to sprint 3.7 miles using about 1,000 pedal revolutions.

These 1,000 pedal revolutions place significant overload on the major leg muscles, such as the hamstrings, quadriceps, and calf. This stress placed on the legs is the likely explanation for the significant increase in muscle mass that we found in our three studies. (See table 4, page 49.) Women increased their leg muscle mass by 0.4 pounds, whereas men increased theirs by 1.1 pounds.

	Light	Moderate	Hard
Pedal rate sprinting	90 rpm	115 rpm	125 rpm
Pedal rate recovery	50 rpm	75 rpm	85 rpm
Pedal resistance	1.1 pounds	2.2 pounds	3.3 pounds
Distance sprinted	2.7 miles	3.4 miles	3.7 miles
Distance recovery	2.2 miles	3.4 miles	3.8 miles
Total distance	4.9 miles	6.8 miles	7.5 miles
Total sprint cycles	720	920	1000
Average sprint power output per 8-second sprint	45 watts	115 watts	188 watts

Table 6. Sample pedal rates and distances cycled for an eight-second-sprint/twelve-second-recovery protocol for twenty minutes at light, moderate, and hard intensities

However, in all three studies, the biggest increase in muscle mass was found in the core muscle area, which includes the rectus abdominis, external and internal obliques, and transverse abdominis. These muscles contract isometrically during sprinting to provide a platform from which to turn over the legs quickly. (Isometric muscle contraction occurs when a muscle is contracted but does not change its length.) In our three studies, both women and men had significant increases in these core muscles, with 0.9 pounds for the women and 1.5 pounds for the men. This increase in muscle mass after cycle interval sprinting is very important because, as mentioned earlier, it has been estimated that each 2.2 pound increase in muscle mass brings an increase of daily energy burning of about 21 calories. If this muscle mass increase was maintained for a year, it would likely increase energy expenditure by about 7,665 calories, which would be equal to burning about 2.2 pounds of fat. A calorie is a measure of energy. Energy is required for our bodies to function during sleep, at rest, and when exercising. The number of calories in food indicates its amount of potential energy. The workout that the leg muscles receive is likely to be the major reason why all studies that have examined cycle interval sprinting and glucose metabolism have shown that it reduces insulin resistance. This finding has major implications for the preventing of type 2 diabetes, which has been shown to be a disease of the legs and liver, in contrast to the arms, which typically do not become insulin resistant.

SPRINT ROWING

Rowing on a stationary rowing machine is a good form of interval sprinting exercise. This exercise is also non-weight-bearing but involves more muscles than cycling, as it uses the upper body too. However, since the limbs do not move as quickly as in cycling, it isn't clear how sprint rowing will affect belly fat. Young adults performing interval sprint rowing in our laboratory have easily boosted their heart rates to similar levels as those generated on the stationary bike, so it is likely that sprint rowing induces significant elevations in catecholamines. Studies measuring the catecholamine response to sprint rowing, however, need to be performed.

SPRINT WALKING

Sprint walking can utilize fast-twitch muscle fibers but probably not to the same extent as cycling. Skeletal muscles contain fast-, intermediate-, and slow-twitch fibers. Slow-twitch fibers are typically activated during walking whereas the intermediate- and fast-twitch fibers are recruited during sprinting. Walking is a reasonable form of exercise for those who like to walk, but it is very difficult to get a young adult's heart rate over 130 beats per minute when sprint walking. Therefore, it is unlikely that sprint walking will produce significant reductions in belly fat.

SPRINT STAIR CLIMBING

Sprint stair climbing is a good form of interval sprinting, as it is possible to get your heart rate over 130 beats per minute. The advantages of stair climbing are that it doesn't expose you to pollution and traffic, and it is inexpensive and time efficient. Stair climbing is a low-impact exercise, although descending is harder on the joints than ascending.

The recommended posture is to keep a straight back, to avoid extending the knees, and to place your entire foot on the step. You should ensure that the staircase you choose is well ventilated and lit, has an even surface, and offers good personal safety. We recommend that you wear cross-trainers rather than running shoes. The net energy cost in calories of stair climbing when walking has been estimated to be about 0.15 calories per 7.9-inch step for a 154-pound male. This is about 1 calorie for 7 steps. The optimal stair-climbing walking rate has been estimated to be 90 steps per minute, so for 270 steps—three minutes of climbing—the energy cost is just below 40 calories. Coming down the stairs burns about a third of the energy as going up. Going up and down for a thousand steps per day would use up about 143 calories.

Stair-climbing programs typically take about twelve minutes a day and are usually split into three four-minute sessions. Interval sprint stair climbing could include an eight-second stair climb followed by a one-minute toning exercise such as push-ups and sit-ups.

SPRINT RUNNING

Sprint running is another form of interval sprinting exercise. It is possible for experienced runners to do it on a treadmill; however, this is a high-risk exercise. Because a treadmill is not able to accelerate and decelerate quickly enough for the eight-second/twelve-second protocol, you have to set the treadmill to sprinting speed and then jump off the treadmill while holding on to the side bars for the twelve-second recovery phase before jumping back on to sprint.

Sounds too dangerous? Then try it on a running track.

Sprint for eight seconds and then easy jog for twelve seconds. Do this continuously around the track. If you don't have a track nearby, you can try sprint running on a flat, grassy surface. Map out a triangle and sprint for eight seconds on one side of the triangle, and then easy jog for twelve seconds on the other two sides. This is probably the hardest type of interval sprinting; for some people, it will place too much stress on their ankle and hip joints.

SPRINT ARM ERGOMETRY

Upper-body interval sprinting training involves rapid movement of the arms. No research to date has investigated the effect of upper-body interval sprinting on muscle adaptations or clinical markers such as blood and muscle lactate. It is likely, however, that this form of exercise will bring about fewer positive changes than lower-body interval sprinting will. Moving the arms rapidly can be achieved by a number of exercise modalities, although the most efficient is the stationary arm ergometer, a piece of equipment similar to a stationary cycle.

SPRINT BOXING

Boxing, especially with a partner, is another form of upper-body interval sprinting exercise. You can do this by yourself if you have access to a punching bag. Your partner can also hold a foam impact pillow while you punch continuously for eight seconds. During the recovery phase, you can shadowbox slowly for twelve seconds—for example, by slow ducking and weaving. Heart rates during this form of exercise can easily get up to 150 beats per minute for young adults; thus, boxing may result in reduced belly fat, but as mentioned, the ability of methods other than cycling to reduce belly fat is undetermined.

SPRINT SKIPPING

Skipping rope is a good form of interval sprinting exercise that you can do by yourself or with a partner. You will need a skipping rope, a suitable surface, and quality footwear. Sprint skip for eight seconds and then easy jog on the spot for twelve seconds. Heart rates during this form of exercise also can easily get up to 150 beats per minute for young adults.

would tomatoes
consequence

SPRINT SWIMMING
instead thraw

Interval sprinting can be done in a swimming pool or in the ocean. A major limitation is timing the sprints or listening to sprint music. It would be possible with waterproof headphones, but counting the seconds as you sprint and recover is also an option. An example would be to sprint using freestyle for eight seconds and then switch to an easy breaststroke for a twelve-second recovery period. It is difficult for nonathletes to get their heart rates up to 150 beats per minute while swimming; therefore, it is unlikely that sprint swimming will result in a significant increase in catecholamines and, consequently, a reduction in belly fat. Research examining the ability of sprint swimming to burn fat, however, needs to be conducted.

INTERVAL SPRINTING CIRCUITS

Interval sprinting circuit training is an excellent form of exercise that you can do by yourself, with a partner, or in a group. Choose a combination of interval sprinting exercises from those listed above; for example, a good whole-body workout could include five minutes of boxing, five minutes of sprint skipping, five minutes of sprint rowing, and five minutes of sprint cycling.

If you have time, it is possible to extend the twenty-minute session by adding a resistance exercise between each sprinting exercise. For example, you could do thirty seconds of push-ups, dips, crunches, biceps curls, lunges, and so forth.

Monitoring Your Progress

To monitor your progress, you need to record a certain amount of information, such as:

- heart-rate response during sprinting exercise;
- heart-rate response during the cool-down;
- pedal rate during bike sprinting exercise;
- pedal resistance during bike sprinting exercise;
- weight and/or body fat change;

- waist circumference change;

- abdominal width change;

- waist skinfold site change;

- lower- and upper-leg circumference changes;

- rating of perceived exertion during exercise; and

- aerobic fitness change, as assessed by a submaximal fitness test.

Heart rate, pedal rate, and pedal resistance have been previously described in this chapter, whereas body composition was outlined in chapter 1. Rating of perceived exertion (RPE) is an easy but effective way of monitoring exercise intensity and has been used to prescribe exercise intensity in a variety of sporting activities and clinical settings. (See appendix D, page 189.)

Aerobic fitness change can be estimated by a submaximal fitness test (see appendix B, page 185), which requires a stationary bike, a heart-rate monitor, and an RPE scale. The test lasts only about ten minutes with a four-minute cooldown and can be performed every month to assess exercise heart-rate change. Three bike protocols for unfit, moderately fit, and highly fit individuals are described on pages 100 to 101. Simply perform the exercise protocol as described, and record your heart rate and RPE at the end of each exercise stage. As can be seen, this submaximal test involves a four-minute warm-up, an easy three-minute cycling stage, a medium-hard three-minute cycling stage, and a moderately hard three-minute cycling stage. The test should not be too tiring, and it is important that your exercise heart rate does not go too high.

After you have finished the test, you should have your resting and exercise heart rates recorded, together with your RPE at the three stages. You can then plot these data on the graph included in appendix C (page 188). You should see your heart rates increase during the three stages after the warm-up. If you are nervous and consequently have a high resting heart rate, your heart rate for stages one and two may be similar. When people get accustomed to the test, however, they typically see a consistent rise in their heart rate across the three stages.

Our laboratory analyzed the heart-rate responses to submaximal exercise from the three interval training studies we'd conducted. We found that a decrease in the average heart rate by 1 beat at stages two and three equalled an increase in aerobic fitness of about 1 percent. Thus, after doing interval sprinting for six weeks, if the average heart rate at stages two and three was lowered by 4 beats per minute, the increase in aerobic fitness would be about 4 percent. Your heart rate will continue to decrease, and you will get fitter, if you either increase your pedal rate or resistance over the following weeks of exercise. For example, an average decrease in heart rate of 10 beats per minute for stages two and three equates to an increase in aerobic fitness of about 10 percent; a decrease of twenty beats per minute, about 20 percent; and so on.

The lowered heart rate during exercise reflects adaptations

in the heart, the muscles, and the blood. It is not possible to have an increase in aerobic fitness without a lowering of heart rate at the same bike power outputs. A monitoring form to record all this information is included in appendix F (page 194). You can copy the form and record this information every week for six weeks. Other information can be recorded on the weekly progress form in appendix G (page 195).

On the following pages are examples of a morning, lunchtime, and evening interval sprinting weekly program, performed at light, moderate, and hard interval sprinting intensities. You should select the method and exercise intensity that is best for you. You might also choose to exercise two mornings per week and once at lunchtime or in the evening.

What about exercising on the other days? It is likely that performing more interval sprinting exercise, either by lengthening each session—say, from twenty minutes to thirty minutes—or by including more sessions, such as adding twenty minutes of interval sprinting on a Sunday, will result in greater adaptations, such as reduced belly fat, increased aerobic fitness, decreased insulin resistance, and increased leg and trunk muscle mass.

	Before sprinting	Time of day: 6:00 a.m. to 8:00 a.m.	Pedal rate and resistance	Information recorded
Monday	Drink water or green tea	20 minutes of LifeSprints	90 rpm at 1.1 pounds, 50 rpm recovery	Weight and fat, exercise heart rate, and RPE
Wednesday	Drink water or green tea	20 minutes of LifeSprints	90 rpm at 1.1 pounds, 50 rpm recovery	Exercise heart rate and RPE
Friday	Drink water or green tea	20 minutes of LifeSprints	90 rpm at 1.1 pounds, 50 rpm recovery	Exercise heart rate and RPE

Table 7. A morning workout (light)

	Before sprinting	Time of day: 12:00 p.m. to 2:00 p.m.	Pedal rate and resistance	Information recorded
Monday	Fast for 2–3 hours and drink water or green tea	20 minutes of LifeSprints	115 rpm at 2.2 pounds, 75 rpm recovery	Weight and fat, exercise heart rate, and RPE
Wednesday	Fast for 2–3 hours and drink water or green tea	20 minutes of LifeSprints	115 rpm at 2.2 pounds, 75 rpm recovery	Exercise heart rate and RPE
Friday	Fast for 2–3 hours and drink water or green tea	20 minutes of LifeSprints	115 rpm at 2.2 pounds, 75 rpm recovery	Exercise heart rate and RPE

Table 8. A lunchtime workout (moderate)

	Before sprinting	Time of day: 6:00 p.m. to 8:00 p.m.	Pedal rate and resistance	Information recorded
Monday	Fast for 2–3 hours after evening meal and drink water or green tea	20 minutes of LifeSprints	125 rpm at 3.3 pounds, 85 rpm recovery	Weight and fat, exercise heart rate, and RPE
Wednesday	Fast for 2–3 hours after evening meal and drink water or green tea	20 minutes of LifeSprints	125 rpm at 3.3 pounds, 85 rpm recovery	Exercise heart rate and RPE
Friday	Fast for 2–3 hours after evening meal and drink water or green tea	20 minutes of LifeSprints	125 rpm at 3.3 pounds, 85 rpm recovery	Exercise heart rate and RPE

Table 9. An evening workout (hard)

*

This chapter has described interval sprinting techniques and modalities. The key points to remember are:

- For best results, it's important to perform interval sprinting correctly by determining your optimal pedal rate and pedal resistance.

- Even if you have a chronic health condition such as heart disease or diabetes, you can participate in interval sprinting. Just be sure to consult your general practitioner or an exercise physiologist before beginning the program.

- It is important to monitor your interval sprinting performance and the health changes that are likely to occur with regular interval sprinting, so that you can measure the amount of belly fat you lose.

Now that you know how to choose the right equipment for interval sprinting and how to use it to get the most benefit from your program, let's look at adopting an eating plan that enhances your exercise program and helps you lose belly fat.

Chapter 4
Dieting, Nutrients, and Belly Fat

Why We Have Become Overweight

The past fifty years have brought an excess of high-calorie processed food and a significant decrease in physical activity to our lives. Fat-inducing factors of the modern diet include increased consumption of sugar, high levels of saturated fat, increased use of unhealthy vegetable oils, and our eating too little fiber and the healthy fats found in foods such as olive oil, fish oils, avocado, and coconut. Our bodies are very good at storing fat but poor at burning it, because for most of our evolutionary history, we have never been faced with such an abundance of food. What's more, modern processed foods tend to put the body into fat-storage mode as opposed to encouraging cells to burn fat. We're also moving less; most of us sit down all day at our computers. Even our children aren't as active as kids used to be, thanks to a decrease in the amount of physical activity they engage in both at school and as recreation. In the United States, the average child spends seven hours a day using entertainment media such as television, computers, phones, and other electronic devices. As discussed in chapter 5, increased levels of daily stress and reduced quality of sleep also affect fat gain.

To counteract these negative factors of modern living, we need to adapt a healthy eating regimen. The healthiest way of eating is based on consuming lots of fruits and vegetables and little processed food, a diet commonly known as the Mediterranean eating plan.

Our Hunter-Gatherer Genetic Legacy

The agricultural revolution occurred some ten thousand years ago, but human evolution began 2.6 million years earlier, in the Paleolithic period.[1] This means we still carry a relatively unchanged ancient genome, or genetic makeup. Although we live in the twenty-first century, from a genetic perspective, we are Paleolithic people. When hunter-gatherers adopted a diet based on grain, their health degenerated quickly, and this decline in health is prevalent today, as lifestyle-related diseases continue to dominate Westernized and developing nations. We eat highly processed, synthetic foods with one-third as much fiber, half as much polyunsaturated and monounsaturated fats, one-quarter as much fish, 60 percent to 70 percent more saturated fat, three times more protein, and up to five times more salt and sugar. Polyunsaturated and monounsaturated fat are unsaturated fats. "Poly" and "mono" refer to the number of unsaturated chemical bonds they contain. These unsaturated fats are typically found

How's your diet?

Use this questionnaire to assess your general diet and find out what changes you might need to make to help reduce the amount of belly fat you carry. Answer the questions below with regard to your typical eating patterns by filling in a score between 1 and 4 for each question and then add up your total.

1 = Not at all   2 = Sometimes

3 = Fairly regularly   4 = All the time

1. I eat junk food every day

2. I drink at least one soft drink every day

3. I eat sugary food such as cakes
    and sweets daily

4. I eat fried food every day

5. I eat fruit every day*

6. I eat vegetables everyday*

TOTAL

* Reverse the scoring for questions 5 and 6:

4 = Not at all   3 = Sometimes

2 = Fairly regularly   1 = All the time

Interpreting your score:

6 to 9 points: low levels of processed food

10 to 12 points: moderately low levels of processed food

13 to 18 points: moderately high levels of processed food

19 to 24 points: high levels of processed food

in liquid vegetable oils. Our problem is that our DNA has evolved in an environment of food scarcity, yet today we are inundated with inexpensive, processed, unhealthy food. Over centuries, our bodies have become very good at storing fat and until recently had never faced the problem of being overweight. Modern humans typically eat an excess of high-calorie processed food and are unable to use up these extra fat stores.

The Problem with Modern Processed Foods

SUGAR

Weight-inducing factors of the modern diet include increased consumption of sugars in general, and of fructose in particular. Fructose is a simple sugar that does not cause a high rise in blood sugar, so it was once recommended as a substitute for sucrose. Sucrose is a carbohydrate and is a compound of glucose and fructose. Fructose now makes up about 10 percent of the average Western diet. The body needs small amounts of fructose, but too much overwhelms our liver and impairs its ability to metabolize nutrients. As a result, the liver converts this sugar to fat and distributes the fat, in the form of triglyceride, into the circulation. Fruits and vegetables have small amounts of fructose, but food manufacturers also add lots of it to a wide range of foods. Much of this added fructose comes in the form of high-fructose corn syrup, which is very inexpensive. The problem is that fructose does not satisfy our appetite—in fact, it makes us hungry. Food manufacturers know that when they add fructose to a food, people eat a lot more of it. Consequently, excess fructose consumption is associated with fat gain.

Almost all packaged foods have some added sugar, so it is important to examine the nutritional fact panel. Unfortunately, US food labeling is problematic as it is not easy to work out the percentage component of sugar within food. Information on the nutritional fact panel that splits out the different sugars and sweeteners is needed.

Be particularly wary of soft drinks, as they are usually full of fructose, and even fruit juice usually contains a lot of it—minus the healthy nutrients of whole fruit. All soft drinks should be eliminated from your eating plan and fruit juice consumed sparingly. As an example, a cup of chopped tomatoes has about 2.5 grams of fructose; a regular-sized soft drink, about 20 grams; and a supersized cola, about 60 grams.

FAT

The second dangerous aspect of the modern diet is our tendency to eat the wrong kinds of fats. Consuming healthy, monounsaturated fats will boost your body's fat-burning capacity, but eat unhealthy, saturated or polyunsaturated fats, and you will likely gain body fat.

Saturated fat is a hard fat and is contained in butter and meat. A US study conducted on men and women ages fifty-five to seventy-five tried to determine if eating saturated fat contributed to belly fat accumulation. Subjects kept a food diary and underwent MRI to assess their belly fat. Results showed men and women who consumed more than 30 percent of their calories in the form of saturated fat had high levels of belly fat stores.

Vegetable oils are also troublesome, as they are full of polyunsaturated fatty acids that go rancid quickly. During preparation for the market, these oils are typically heated and have solvents added, and they can also be exposed to air and sunlight. This processing destroys their nutritional value and also creates oxidants, which are dangerous for health. Oxidants occur naturally in the human body; however, harmful oxidants, or free radicals, can damage body cells. If free radicals accumulate, they can depress the immune system and cause degenerative disease development. Oils made from canola, corn, safflower, soy, or sunflower are among the most highly refined polyunsaturated products. Also, polyunsaturated oils have been shown to slow down the thyroid gland and thus spur fat gain. You should not heat any vegetable oil. Use coconut oil (a saturated fat), but don't heat it to a temperature higher than 320°F. Coconut oil is full of saturated medium-chain fatty acids. It is unusual among saturated fats because studies have shown that natural coconut oil promotes fat burning, prevents certain diseases, and has antiaging properties. Instead of the medium-chain fatty acids in coconut oil going into the circulation, they travel straight to the liver, where they influence enzyme activity and induce fat burning. In contrast, long-chain fatty acids are typically stored as body fat. Long-chain fatty acids, which make up most of the standard American diet, vary in length from 16 to 24 carbons. In contrast, medium-chain fatty acids are composed of 4 to 14 carbons. Because medium-chain fatty acids have fewer carbon atoms they are healthier than long-chain fatty acids. Medium-chain fatty acids are fat but they are more like carbohydrates and are easy to digest and are more easily burned as energy. Coconut oil is also antibacterial and is very good for the skin. Coconut oil can be used for stir-fries; however, the best way to stir-fry is to use no oil at all. Coconut butter is also an excellent substitute for butter and margarine. You can buy coconut oil in health stores, and there are numerous websites with recipes using coconut oil.[2]

Olive oil is another excellent fat that has proven health benefits. Your olive oil should be as fresh as possible, stored in the fridge, and kept away from sunlight. Buy small bottles and replace them every three to four weeks. Make sure to buy local so that transit time is reduced.

Don't forget about fruits high in antioxidants, such as avocado and papaya. Antioxidants are compounds in foods that negate the effect of free radicals. Free radicals are produced naturally in the body and contribute to the development of heart disease, liver disease, and certain cancers. Fruits, vegetables, whole grains, and nuts contain high levels of antioxidants. Avocado has more fat than any other fruit, and, like olive oil, it is mainly in the form of healthy mono-unsaturated fat. These versatile greenish-purple fruit can be eaten as a snack, as a dip, added to a spicy pasta sauce, or sliced on top of grilled chicken breast. They should be eaten raw. The health benefits of avocado include contributing to the prevention of arthritis, dementia, heart disease, and type

2 diabetes. Papaya, too, is eaten raw, but squeezing a slice of lemon or lime over the fruit enhances its natural flavor. Consuming papaya has been shown to help reduce the incidence of atherosclerosis, colon cancer, type 2 diabetes, and macular disease of the eye.

Finally, omega-3 polyunsaturated fatty acids, found primarily in oily fish, have proven health benefits. Interestingly, it has been estimated that the great majority of people who eat processed food diets are typically omega-3 deficient. Omega-3s in the diet can protect against cardiovascular heart disease, lower blood lipids, increase vascular function, and decrease inflammation.[3] The main chemicals in omega-3s that are thought to enhance health are eicosapentaenoic (EPA) and docosahexaenoic (DHA) acids. A number of plants and vegetables contain EPA and DHA, such as Chinese broccoli, flaxseed, and spinach, but the highest amounts are contained in oily fish such as tuna, salmon, and mackerel.

PROTEIN

The third dangerous aspect of the modern diet is that we tend to eat too much of the wrong kinds of protein, namely red meat. For years, the food industry has convinced people that we must consume plenty of meat to get all the protein we need to be healthy. Protein, as the advertisements point out correctly, is an essential nutrient, but this emphasis on protein has created the false notion that the only source of protein is from animal products. In Western societies, meals revolve primarily around meat and dairy.

Our obsession with getting enough protein and eating animal products at almost every meal has created a situation of protein overload.[4] In fact, all plant foods contain protein, and it is possible to get all the protein you need from a strict vegetarian diet.[5] Consider the paradox whereby a cow grows quickly from a 44-pound calf to a 750-pound steer simply from eating grass.[6] It doesn't eat chicken or steak to get its protein! Even larger is the African elephant, also a vegetarian.

Eating high levels of animal protein can cause health problems.[7] If we eat too much meat instead of vegetables, we are depriving ourselves of vital plant nutrients. Studies show that people who eat meat face twice the odds of dying from heart disease, are 60 percent more likely to die from cancer, and have a 30 percent greater chance of dying from other lifestyle-related diseases. There is now a plethora of research evidence supporting the health benefits of an unprocessed, plant-based diet. For example, it is now possible to create images of damaged heart arteries using MRI or computed tomography and then show that a plant-based diet reverses atherosclerosis. Ingesting meat proteins increases blood cholesterol levels to a greater extent than consuming saturated fat. When diets of different countries are compared, results have shown that people consuming traditional plant-based diets experience significantly lower incidences of heart disease. In Westernized countries, people who eat more plant-based foods also are less likely to develop heart disease. Vegetables such as asparagus, cauliflower, spinach, mung beans, and broccoli pack high levels of protein.[8] Nuts, too, are a great source of both protein and healthy fats. Almonds, hazelnuts, brazil nuts, and cashews are all excellent sources of nutrition and are great to snack on when you feel hungry between meals. All nuts should be raw and free from additives such as salt.

FIBER

The fourth dangerous aspect of the modern diet is that we tend to eat too little fiber. Fiber is that portion of food that cannot be digested by enzymes in the human digestive tract, and so it does not provide any nutrients. But fiber plays a key role in regulating bowel activity. Nutritionists recommend that we eat at least 30 grams of fiber daily; unfortunately, most people in Western cultures consume only about half this amount. Importantly, all fruits and vegetables contain more fiber than processed foods. High-fiber fruits include apples, blackberries, pears, and raspberries, while fiber-rich vegetables include broccoli, Brussels sprouts, chickpeas, lentils, and lima beans.

Fiber was first found to be important when physicians working in Africa noticed that the native people there who remained on traditional diets enjoyed very good health, but when they began eating refined grains and sugars, their health deteriorated. This discovery became known as the fiber hypothesis.

Studies have shown that men and women who consume the most fiber have the lowest incidence of colorectal cancer. It has been estimated that if Americans increased their fiber intake by 13 grams a day from food sources—not from supplements—about a third of the 131,607 cases of colorectal cancers diagnosed each year could be avoided. However, it is not clear if this protective effect is due solely to high-fiber foods, because people whose diets are rich in fiber typically eat less meat. What is clear, however, is that diets naturally high in fiber and low in animal foods can prevent colon cancer.

The Effects of Dieting on Belly Fat and Skeletal Muscle

Severe dieting, such as cutting down the amount of food you eat by half, has been shown to produce weight loss in the short term, but most of the pounds dropped are in the form of body water and muscle protein. Some fat is typically lost, but *keeping it off* is harder than losing it in the first place. Of those who lose body fat from drastic diets, over 90 percent will put the fat back on within five years.[9]

Furthermore, a number of unhealthy consequences accompany severe dieting. The major problem is that cutting your daily calories in half for weeks or months will cause significant decreases in muscle mass. Skeletal muscle is very important for health and is one of the major tissues involved in fat burning; as mentioned, 2.2 pounds of muscle mass has the potential to burn up to an extra 6.6 pounds of fat per year. Other potential adverse effects from severe dieting include a reduced intake of essential minerals, vitamins, and proteins, though these malnutrition aspects depend on the nature of the diet. Low-fat diets may also deprive individuals of healthy fats such as the polyunsaturated or monounsaturated fats found in fish, olives, avocados, and coconuts.

The five major problems with severe dieting are:

- a loss of muscle mass;

- reduced vitamins and minerals;

- a decrease in body water rather than body fat;

- reduced energy and increased fatigue; and

- constant hunger.

When it comes to belly fat and dieting, studies have shown that belly fat is easier to lose than subcutaneous fat. However, if you only cut the amount of calories you consume and don't exercise, you will lose some belly fat in the first two to three weeks, but after that, your progress will plateau.[10] The diets evaluated in these studies have typically been starvation diets. Thus, the majority of diets, irrespective of their nature, are not sustainable in the long term, either because they are deficient nutritionally or because they provide little in the way of variety, are difficult to carry out, and expensive. What is needed instead is an eating plan that does not involve counting calories or starving yourself. Eating plans should be healthy but at the same time be fun and sustainable. A balanced eating plan should contain little junk food and processed food; small amounts of red meat, good fats, and carbohydrates; and lots of plant protein. We recommend the Mediterranean eating plan.

The Mediterranean Eating Plan to Help Reduce Belly Fat

The Mediterranean eating plan is closely tied to areas of olive cultivation. However, it works to improve health even if you don't happen to live in that part of the world.[11] The diet involves eating lots of fruits and vegetables, beans, bread, nuts, whole grain cereals, fish, and seeds. White meat, such as free-range chicken and fish, is eaten occasionally, and red meat sparingly. Good fats—coconut oil, olive oil, and omega-3s (fish oil)—are consumed instead of saturated animal fat. Processed food is rarely eaten. You're allowed moderate amounts of wine, usually with meals, and dark chocolate, a good source of antioxidants. Junk food and fried food are eliminated.

The cardioprotective effects of omega-3 fatty acids, polyphenols, oleic acid, natural antioxidants, and folic acid, all plentiful in the Mediterranean eating plan, have been demonstrated.[12] Polyphenols are antioxidants whereas oleic acid is a monounsaturated fatty acid found naturally in plant sources and animal products. Folic acid is a B-group vitamin that is important for healthy fetal development. Consuming foods rich in arginine, an amino acid found in nuts and fish, has been associated with decreased inflammation. High-fiber diets have also been associated with lowered inflammation levels. Inflammation is part of the body's immune response to something that enters or irritates our bodies. Inflammation often occurs when we pick up a bacterium or virus, or when we injure a joint in an accident or sporting injury. Inflammation can also occur in overweight people who get little exercise and eat lots of processed food.

Inflammation is detrimental to our health; it has been found that people with coronary artery disease typically have high levels of inflammation. Inflammation is typically assessed by measuring blood levels of inflammatory chemicals called cytokines such as C-reactive protein and interleukin-6. Olive oil is rich in medium-chain fatty acids, which improve blood fat profiles and reduce cardiovascular risk by decreasing the amount of low-density lipoprotein (LDL, the "bad" form of cholesterol) in the blood, while enhancing the level of "good" high-density lipoprotein (HDL) cholesterol. Medium-chain fatty acid intake has also been shown to lower concentrations of insulin and glucose.

How the Mediterranean eating plan works is unclear, but the fruits, vegetables, and nuts contain lots of phytonutrients high in antioxidant and folic acid levels. Phytonutrients are nutrients derived from plants and are essential for sustaining human life.

There are also significant health benefits from consuming healthy fats such as monounsaturated olive oil and the poly-unsaturated omega-3s contained in fish oils.

How to Calculate Your Mediterranean Eating Score

Some people will have a number of Mediterranean foods already in their current diet, so it is useful to assess how much Mediterranean food you are eating. This can be done by calculating your Mediterranean eating score by filling in the table on page 118.

To use the table, write a score in the right-hand column that reflects your typical diet. For the beneficial components, if you eat more than the average per day, your score is 1. For example, consuming more than 500 grams of vegetables per day gives you a score of 1. If you eat less than 500 grams of vegetables, your score is 0. For the detrimental components, if you eat less than the average, your score is 1. For example, 90 grams or less of meat per day gives you a 1. If you eat more than 90 grams of meat, then your score is 0.

Studies have shown that people experience significant health benefits after improving their score from 2 to 4, so health can be enhanced without having to achieve a perfect Mediterranean eating plan score of 8.

Mediterranean Food

When cooking the Mediterranean way, grilling and boiling are the preferred methods.

BEANS, PEAS, AND PASTAS

Beans contain lots of fiber, protein, healthy carbohydrates, and iron. Most beans are also good sources of magnesium, which is important for heart health, and calcium, which is essential for bone health. Healthy beans and peas include black-eyed peas, chickpeas, green peas, lentils, snow peas, and black, kidney, lima, pinto, and navy beans.

Beans contain almost no fat and are low in calories. Sometimes called legumes, beans are one of the best plant

Diet component			
Beneficial components	Average (per day)	The Mediterranean eating plan recommends	Score
Vegetables	500 grams	5 average-sized servings	
Legumes	7 grams	1 cup	
Fruits and nuts	360 grams	4 pieces of fruit and a handful of nuts	
Cereals	140 grams	1 bowl of cereal	
Monounsaturated: saturated fat ratio	1:7		
Detrimental components	Average (per day)	The Mediterranean eating plan recommends	Score
Meat and poultry	90 grams	Less than 1 chicken breast	
Dairy products	190 grams	Less than 1 glass of milk and 1 yogurt	
Alcohol consumption *14.4 ounces in a schooner and 19.3 ounces in a pint	5 to 25 grams	Less than 2 schooners of beer*	

Adapted from Trichopoulou et al.(2003).[13]

Interpreting your score:

0 to 2 points: low levels of Mediterranean eating

3 to 4 points: moderately low levels of Mediterranean eating

5 to 6 points: moderately high levels of Mediterranean eating

7 to 8 points: high levels of Mediterranean eating

sources of protein, fiber, and iron. Because they contain high levels of protein, a single serving can suppress your appetite for hours. Beans can also contribute to your daily fiber requirements. For example, there are approximately 8 grams of fiber in a half cup of cooked lentils, which amounts to about 25 percent of your daily fiber needs. Unfortunately, most canned beans contain high levels of salt in the form of sodium. Check the nutrition label to make sure you buy only unsalted beans. Alternatively, buy dried beans and soak them according to packet instructions before cooking them.

Most pastas and noodles are full of simple carbohydrates (refined sugars) and have little nutritional value. Also, processed pasta and noodles are treated with a chlorine dioxide bleach that destroys most nutrients. Overprocessed noodles and pasta should be replaced with pasta and noodles such as wholemeal pasta, spelt pasta, rice pasta, kamut pasta, quinoa pasta, ramen noodles, soba noodles, and udon noodles.

BEVERAGES

The Mediterranean eating plan permits one glass of alcohol per day for women and two for men. All alcohol appears to have health benefits if drunk in moderation.[14] Avoid sugary soft drinks and fruit juices, as they contain refined sources of sugars, especially fructose. Replace soft drinks with water, green tea, or coffee, which all have proven health benefits.

CHOCOLATE

Dark chocolate and cocoa powder contain numerous antioxidants and high amounts of iron. One cup of cocoa powder provides about two-thirds of daily iron requirements. In contrast, a typical chocolate bar contains only about 6 percent cocoa, so it is important to buy quality dark chocolate that consists of at least 70 percent cocoa if you need to satisfy a chocolate craving.

DAIRY PRODUCTS

Low to moderate amounts of dairy foods, such as cheese, milk, and yogurt, are allowed on the Mediterranean eating plan. Low-fat or fat-free dairy foods should be used instead of full-fat versions.

FATS

The main fat used in the Mediterranean eating plan is olive oil. Make sure to buy virgin or extra-virgin products. Olive oil undergoes minimal processing, so it retains its healthy plant antioxidants. In contrast, most other polyunsaturated oils, such as canola, safflower, and corn, are heated and treated with solvents to improve their shelf life and appearance, which decreases their healthy plant compounds.

FRUITS

Fruits are healthy and taste delicious. They contain lots of vitamins A and C and other health-supporting nutrients.

People who eat four to five portions of fruit each day have low levels of heart disease, stroke, and hypertension. Although the vitamins in fruit promote health, taking these exact vitamins in the form of supplements does not appear to enhance health as much. Fruit also contains fiber, minerals, and antioxidants that work synergistically to protect against lifestyle-related diseases. All fruits are healthy, but the following are nutrient dense and appear to have the most disease-fighting potential: apples, avocados, bananas, blueberries, grapes, kiwis, oranges, papaya, and strawberries. Other healthy fruits typically consumed on the Mediterranean eating plan are cherries, dates, peaches, grapefruit, and melon, most of which contain high levels of vitamin C.

The majority of fruits have similar amounts of glucose and fructose. Apples and pears, however, contain more fructose than glucose. Fructose needs glucose to help it exit the small intestine and enter the portal vein to arrive in the liver. Therefore, people who eat a lot of apples and pears end up with fructose remaining in their small intestine. Some people are fructose intolerant, and for them this causes bacteria to colonize the bowel, triggering abdominal pain and discomfort. To test if you are fructose intolerant, stop eating apples and pears and drinking fruit juice and soft drinks for two weeks and see if the symptoms go away. If they do, then you are likely to be fructose intolerant.

You should try to eat fresh fruits as much as possible. Unfortunately, the nutritional value of fruit can diminish rapidly if they sit out for days or did not arrive fresh to the supermarket. Chemicals such as pesticides are also used in fruit and vegetable farming to increase production, although most developed countries restrict the amounts allowed in foods to levels that are considered safe. Pesticides are still toxic chemicals that kill agricultural pests, however, and they can cause health problems for people if consumed in large amounts. If you want to avoid pesticides, buy organic food grown without the use of chemicals and pesticides or wash fruits and veggies thoroughly using liquid cleansers.

NUTS AND SEEDS

Nuts and seeds are another important part of the Mediterranean eating plan. About 80 percent of the calories in nuts come from fat, although the majority of that fat is unsaturated. Nuts are high in calories, so try not to eat more than a handful per day. Healthy nuts include raw almonds, Brazil nuts, cashews, pine nuts, hazelnuts, peanuts, pistachios, and macadamias. Seeds, from pumpkin, sesame, sunflower, and flax, are also full of iron and other phytonutrients. A number of nutrients in nuts work synergistically to enhance health. These include fats that lower blood cholesterol, fiber and plant sterols that reduce cholesterol reabsorption, arginine, which helps retain blood vessel elasticity, antioxidant vitamins and minerals that reduce inflammation, and low sodium and high potassium levels, which help maintain a normal blood pressure. All nuts and seeds should be unsalted and eaten raw.

POULTRY AND RED MEAT

Neither poultry nor red meat should be consumed in high amounts when on the Mediterranean eating plan. Ideally, limit red meat to one or two meals per month. Although poultry appears to be healthier than red meat, it depends on whether you are getting your chicken from a free range or a factory farm. Chickens reared on factory farms are abused animals, typically packed by the thousands into massive, crowded sheds. They are fed large amounts of antibiotics and drugs to keep them alive, and these antibiotics make chickens grow large at an abnormally fast rate. You only have to go to the supermarket and compare the size of a free-range chicken with a factory-farm chicken to realize that something is wrong. A free-range chicken is always much smaller because it is not receiving antibiotics or being fed nutrients that increase its growth. If you want to eat chicken, make sure it is free range. Chicken is a good source of protein, but you can treat yourself to much healthier forms of protein by eating vitamin- and iron-rich beans, legumes, seeds, and grains.

SEAFOOD

When on the Mediterranean eating plan, you should consume two servings of fish or shellfish per week in place of red meat and poultry. Choices include: flounder, lobster, mackerel, mussels, oysters, prawn, salmon, squid, and tuna.

SEASONING AND SPREADS

In the Mediterranean eating plan, spices replace salt for seasoning. Try sprinkling food with chillies, cinnamon, cloves, garlic, ginger, paprika, parsley, sage, saffron, and turmeric.

Two herbs that can be used to replace salt are garlic powder and freshly ground (not preground) black pepper. Other options include onion powder (not onion salt). Butter and margarine are not used on the Mediterranean eating plan; you can replace them with coconut butter or nut butter.

VEGETABLES

Vegetables are a good source of protein, fiber, vitamin C, beta-carotene, calcium, and folic acid. Beta-carotene is a red, orange, or yellow pigment and is called a carotenoid. Beta-carotene and other carotenoids provide about half of the vitamin A required in the American diet. It is found in fruits, vegetables, and whole grains. Vegetables are low in calories yet high in nutrition. All vegetables are cholesterol free, and nearly all contain no saturated fat; those vegetables that do contain fat usually have it in small amounts of healthy unsaturated fat. The energy in vegetables comes from complex carbohydrate. As its name suggests, this sugar takes much more time to digest than simple carbohydrate, and consequently results in much lower blood levels of glucose and insulin. However, some vegetables have a high glycemic index, which means that, when eaten, they trigger high concentrations of sugar and insulin in the circulation. High-glycemic vegetables include beetroot and corn.

The Mediterranean diet calls for eating five to seven servings of vegetables every day. If you reduce your consumption of red meat, then you should eat vegetables that are high in iron and vitamin C to prevent a deficiency of red blood cells, a condition known as anemia. Vegetables containing high levels of iron are cooked Swiss chard, cooked turnip greens, raw kale, and raw beetroot greens, whereas those high in vitamin C are broccoli, red and green chillies, capsicum, fresh thyme and parsley, and dark, leafy vegetables such as kale and cress. Other healthy vegetables typically consumed on the Mediterranean eating plan are artichokes, celery, eggplant, lettuce, onions, peas, peppers, mushrooms, sweet potatoes, and tomatoes. You should try to eat fresh vegetables whenever possible. As with fruits, veggies' nutritional value falls the longer they sit on the shelf. The good news is that frozen vegetables and canned fruits contain about the same amount of healthy nutrients as when they are fresh.

WHOLE GRAINS

The grains that you eat should be whole grains that contain no saturated or trans fat. Trans fats are unhealthy unsaturated fats that act like saturated fats. Consumption of trans fats increases heart disease risk by elevating low-density lipoprotein cholesterol and lowering high-density lipoprotein cholesterol in the blood. Whole grains typically consumed on the Mediterranean eating plan are oats, barley, buckwheat, bulgur wheat, couscous, millet, and rice. All these grains are rich in iron.

It is best not to eat processed cereals, as they are nutritionally poor, typically containing high levels of sugar in the form of fructose. If you have to eat a commercial breakfast cereal, check its nutrition facts panel first.

Sample Recipes for a Mediterranean Breakfast, Lunch, and Dinner

There are hundreds of Mediterranean recipes and cooking tips available on recipe websites such as *EatingWell* (www.eatingwell.com), and an extensive number of healthy Mediterranean recipes are also to be found in books like *UltraMetabolism* by Dr. Mark Hyman and *The Complete Idiot's Guide to Belly Fat Weight Loss* by Claire Wheeler and Diane A. Welland. Below you'll find a sample menu of recipes suitable for breakfast, lunch, and dinner. Each recipe serves one person, unless stated otherwise.

Breakfast

SCRAMBLED EGGS AND TOAST

A good Mediterranean breakfast is scrambled eggs on whole grain toast. Butter or margarine should not be used on the toast. Going without butter may be difficult, but coconut or nut butter can be used as a healthy substitute. This meal can be followed by whole fruit such as an orange or a slice of melon. Drink unsweetened Sencha green tea, black tea, coffee, or water; do not drink fruit juice, as it contains high concentrations of fructose.

You will need:

2 eggs

1 tablespoon low-fat or skim milk

1 teaspoon freshly ground black pepper or spice of your choice

Method

1. Beat the eggs with the milk and freshly ground black pepper.

2. Pour mixture into a heated nonstick fry pan and scramble until done.

3. Serve scrambled eggs on whole grain toast.

FRUIT, NUTS, AND YOGURT

This breakfast is quick to prepare and can contain a range of fruit and nuts. The yogurt should be nonfat or low-fat Greek.

You will need:

½ cup to 1 cup fruit of your choice, such as banana, melon, berries, mango, apple, or pear

½ cup low-fat, low-sugar, or sugar-free yogurt

½ cup raw, unsalted nuts of your choice, such as almonds, cashews, or hazelnuts, chopped

Method

1. Chop larger fruit into smaller pieces, but keep fruit whole whenever possible. Place fruit in a cereal bowl.

2. Cover fruit with yogurt. Sprinkle chopped raw nuts over the yogurt.

CEREAL AND FRUIT (SERVES 2)

As most commercial cereals contain lots of sugar, it is best if you make your own. Adding blueberries, chopped bananas, and peaches to a healthy homemade cereal creates a great breakfast. Use low-fat milk, but if you don't like cow's milk, try a nondairy milk such as coconut, rice, or soy. If you don't want any milk, add fresh fruit and yogurt.

Dr. Stephen Boutcher

You will need:

2 tablespoons sunflower seeds

4 tablespoons sliced almonds

2 tablespoons nuts of your choice, such as almonds, cashews, or hazelnuts, chopped

1½ cups rolled oats

2 tablespoons sultanas or your preferred dried fruit

1 teaspoon cinnamon

Method

1. Place sunflower seeds, sliced almonds, chopped nuts, and rolled oats in a bowl and mix well.

2. To sweeten, add the sultanas and cinnamon.

3. Serve with low-fat milk or yogurt and top with the fruit of your choice.

Lunch

CURRIED VEGETABLES

Any vegetable can be used in this recipe; however, harder vegetables such as carrots and potatoes should be precooked.

You will need:

1 tablespoon olive oil

1 cup mixed vegetables such as asparagus, onions, potatoes, carrots, broccoli, peas, and capsicum, chopped

2 eggs

1 teaspoon curry powder

Method

1. Place olive oil in a frying pan over medium heat. Add vegetables and stir-fry for 3 minutes.

2. Beat the eggs in a bowl and add curry powder.

3. Add eggs to the vegetables and cook for 3 minutes, stirring occasionally until the eggs are cooked.

SPICY BURRITO (SERVES 4)

Beans are extremely healthy (if you buy the canned, salt-free variety) and quick to prepare. Multiple toppings can be used to generate many different flavors, and this burrito can be spiced up by adding chili powder and cayenne pepper.

You will need:

1 tablespoon olive oil

1 onion, chopped

1 red capsicum, chopped

14-ounce can salt-free kidney beans or mixed beans

1 clove garlic, crushed

¼ teaspoon chili powder

¼ teaspoon cayenne pepper

½ cabbage, shredded

1 tomato, diced, seeds removed

½ red onion, diced

1 teaspoon coriander, chopped

1 teaspoon lime juice

freshly ground black pepper, to taste

1 tablespoon low-fat sour cream

4 tortillas

Method

1. Put olive oil in a frying pan and place over medium heat.

2. Sauté onion and capsicum for 5 minutes, turning occasionally, until soft and onion is transparent.

3. Add beans, garlic, chili powder, and cayenne pepper, and sauté for another 10 minutes.

4. Meanwhile, place cabbage, tomato, red onion, coriander, lime juice, black pepper, and sour cream in a bowl and mix thoroughly. Heat tortillas in the oven.

5. Divide the bean mixture between the tortillas and top with the cabbage salsa; then roll each tortilla to create the burritos.

Dinner

ROASTED SALMON WITH ASPARAGUS

This meal combines healthy salmon with asparagus.

You will need:

2 tablespoons macadamia nuts, crushed

2 tablespoons coriander, chopped

1 tablespoon coconut butter

1 teaspoon lemon zest

6-ounce piece of fresh salmon

freshly ground black pepper, to taste

6 asparagus spears

1 tablespoon olive oil

1 tablespoon Parmesan shavings

Lemon slices, to serve

Method

1. Preheat the oven to 450°F.

2. Combine macadamia nuts and coriander in a bowl. Add the coconut butter and lemon zest and mix well.

3. Place salmon on a tray, skin side down, and season with freshly ground black pepper. Spread macadamia and coriander mix thickly over the salmon flesh. Place in the oven and roast for 12 to 16 minutes, until just cooked.

4. While your salmon is roasting, preheat the grill to medium. Place asparagus spears on a baking tray, drizzle with olive oil, and place under the grill for 3 to 4 minutes.

5. Place asparagus spears on a plate and cover with Parmesan shavings and freshly ground black pepper. Place the salmon fillet on top of the asparagus spears and garnish with lemon slices.

LEMON CAPER CHICKEN

Serve this meal with sautéed whole greens of your choice.

You will need:

1 small chicken breast, trimmed of all fat

Freshly ground black pepper, to taste

1 clove garlic, crushed

1 tablespoon olive oil

Zest and juice of half a lemon

¼ cup chicken stock

½ cup couscous

¼ cup fresh parsley leaves, chopped

2.3 ounces cherry tomatoes, quartered

1 tablespoon capers, drained

1 spring onion, sliced

Method

1. Place chicken breast, pepper, garlic, and olive oil in a shallow dish and mix together.

2. Heat a medium saucepan over medium-high heat and then add the chicken mixture. Cook for 2 to 3 minutes while tossing the mixture until almost cooked. Transfer to a plate and keep warm by covering the plate with foil.

3. Increase heat to high and add lemon juice and stock. Cook until the liquid comes to a boil and then remove the saucepan and add couscous. Make sure none of the mixture sticks to the bottom of the pan. Cover and let stand for 2 to 3 minutes.

4. Now add the chicken, parsley, tomatoes, capers, onion, and lemon zest. Combine and serve.

How to Switch to the Mediterranean Eating Plan

Beginning the Mediterranean eating plan is simple and will soon become habit if you follow it for six weeks. Replace red meat with white meat, such as fish and free-range chicken, and with tofu. Drink only filtered water and green tea. Cut down saturated fat so that it forms less than 8 percent of your total calories, although you can use coconut oil occasionally, as it is a healthy form of saturated fat. Use the good fats, such as olive oil and those containing omega-3s, more frequently; they should make up about 20 percent to 30 percent of your daily calories. Use a fish oil supplement—one that gives you about 1.8 grams per day is best—if you are not eating lots of fish or seafood or are concerned about toxins such as mercury. Mercury in fish is probably not a health consideration for most people; however, it is an issue for pregnant and breastfeeding women and children up to six years. Replace sweets and sugary foods with fruit and low-fat, low-sugar, or sugar-free yogurt. For example, an orange contains only 77 calories but provides over 4 grams of fiber and lots of other nutrients, such as vitamin C. In contrast, a typical chocolate bar contains no fiber or helpful nutrients but packs about 238 calories—over three times more than the orange. Replace milk chocolate with an extra-fine dark chocolate that has at least 70 percent cocoa, and eat it sparingly. After six weeks, you should have more energy and vitality, and most people won't need to count calories.

Although changing eating habits can be challenging, following the three steps below should increase your chance of converting successfully to a healthy Mediterranean eating plan. And if all this sounds complicated, consult a dietician.

- Identify Mediterranean foods. Read the previous section and seek out more detailed information from the resources mentioned.

- The majority of your eating plan should involve consuming healthy fruits, vegetables, whole grains, nuts, and beans. Processed foods such as French fries and meat, soft drinks, margarine, cakes, and cookies should be eliminated.

• Replace red meat mostly with fish and some free-range chicken and turkey. Limit your consumption of red meat to two portions per month.

How to Keep the Fat Off

Let's say that you lose body fat by adopting the Mediterranean eating plan and the interval sprinting program described in chapter 3. How do you then keep it off? Unfortunately, keeping fat off is more difficult than losing it in the first place. As mentioned, over 90 percent of people who lose body fat by dieting will put it back on again after five years.[15] The difficulty in maintaining body fat loss is that continuing with dieting and exercise is extremely challenging for most men and women. A tiny percentage of people, however, don't regain the fat they've lost. Not much was known about keeping fat off until the National Weight Control Registry (NWCR) was established in the United States in 1994. The NWCR is a database of over five thousand people who have each lost a minimum of 30 pounds of weight and kept it off for at least twelve months. Average weight loss in the NWCR is 66 pounds, and the average period of weight loss is greater than five years.[16] This group of people volunteered to be monitored to help show what really is important for long-term weight control.

The NWCR study discovered that people who were successful in keeping body fat off shared seven healthy habits:

- They had a healthy eating plan

- They exercised regularly.

- They ate breakfast every day.

- They stayed clear of fast food.

- They reduced their energy intake by eating a low-saturated-fat diet.

- They followed a consistent eating plan.

- They reduced their TV watching hours.

As we can see, people who are successful in keeping fat off eat healthily, exercise regularly, and always eat breakfast. An interesting characteristic of the NWCR volunteers was that they ate out less than once per week, on average. The unhealthy effects of most fast foods is well documented, but even in restaurants that serve healthier food, there are still concerns about salt levels and overheating and repeated use of cooking oils. As would be expected, most people in the NWCR followed a low-calorie diet that was also low in saturated fat. Reducing energy intake, however, does not mean eating less food. Staying away from calorie-rich foods allows you to enjoy more of the delicious, healthy dishes contained in a Mediterranean eating plan.

Those who followed a consistent, structured eating plan maintained more weight loss. This is because flexible, spontaneous eating plans offer more opportunities to eat highly processed, unhealthy foods. The NWCR study and a number of others have shown that those who watch a lot of TV are typically overweight. Therefore, substituting some physical activity for TV time is helpful for maintaining fat loss.

Nutrients That Enhance or Impede Fat Burning

Our studies have shown that a person's nutritional patterns when attempting to lose fat through interval sprinting may decrease or enhance fat burning. Some individuals may have an eating plan that includes lots of healthy, unprocessed foods such as fruits, vegetables, and fish, which enhance fat burning, while others may consume soft drinks, sweets, and other processed foods that contain high levels of fructose or other refined products, which suppress fat burning.

Nutrients that enhance fat burning typically affect the fat-burning hormones or their cell receptors. For example, drinking green tea results in enhanced fat burning by blocking enzymes that degrade norepinephrine. Norepinephrine and epinephrine are the major fat-burning hormones and are responsible for releasing fat from fat cells and inducing fat burning in tissues such as the liver and skeletal muscle. A catechin present in green tea called epigallocatechin gallate (EGCG) appears to be responsible for this effect. Catechins are an antioxidant; the highest levels are found in the leaves of the tea plant *Camellia sinensis*. An *American Journal of Clinical Nutrition* article showed that drinking four cups of green tea a day resulted in a loss of more than 6 pounds in eight weeks. However, other clinical trials have not shown a fat-loss effect after green tea consumption. Caffeine, too, induces fat burning, but does so by stimulating the nervous system, which elevates levels of epinephrine in the blood, and by blocking the adenosine receptors on fat cells that suppress fat release. Research has shown that drinking 17 ounces of cold water can increase metabolic rate by a third, mainly due to an increase in fat-releasing hormones such as norepinephrine. Drinking two cups of warm rather than cold water resulted in a much smaller increase in metabolic rate.

Consuming omega-3 fatty acids may also contribute to fat loss by triggering fat-burning enzymes inside cells. Omega-3s also appear to improve leptin signalling in the brain, which reduces appetite. Cold-water fish such as tuna and salmon are good sources of omega-3, as are nuts, seeds, and flaxseed, which contain fats that are changed to omega-3s when ingested.

Capsaicin, the compound that makes chillies hot, has also been shown to enhance fat burning. Most of the research examining the fat-burning effect of chillies has administered the capsaicin in capsule form, which has been found to be more effective than when it's contained in food. The mechanisms underlying the capsaicin effect are unclear but are likely to include an increase in energy expenditure, impeded fat-cell growth, and reduced appetite. Capsaicin can be obtained naturally by consuming raw, cooked, dried, or powdered chillies and capsicums. Cayenne pepper or hot sauce can also be added to homemade soups and meals.

We believe that other nutrients and minerals may enhance or impede fat burning indirectly. For example, having a deficiency of red blood cells is associated with a slower metabolism, resulting in less fat burning. So correcting low red blood cell levels—anemia—can improve the body's ability to burn fat; a cup of lentils provides about 35 percent of daily iron needs.

The thyroid gland affects every cell in the body and has a significant impact on metabolism and fat loss or gain, immunity, hormones, heart rate, and blood pressure. Thyroid dysfunction often has a genetic influence; it isn't unusual for grandparents, parents, and children to all possess thyroid dysfunction. However, nutrients in food can also increase or decrease thyroid function. For example, iodized salt contains iodine, which is essential for thyroid function. Avoiding table salt and consuming little iodine is likely to result in a depressed thyroid in most people. Processed foods typically contain lots of salt, but not the iodized kind. Meat and chicken generally contain antibiotics and growth stimulants that have been shown to reduce thyroid function. Surprisingly, some vegetables impede iodine absorption, reducing thyroid function. Such vegetables usually contain a chemical called goitrogen; however, cooking typically negates this goitrogen effect. Thyroid-reducing vegetables include green, leafy vegetables such as raw cabbage, broccoli, and spinach. Soy also contains goitrogens, and studies have shown that although it is thought of as a healthy food, soy is detrimental for thyroid function; therefore, avoid cooking oils and margarine containing soybean. Replace oils containing soybean with coconut oil and extra-virgin olive oil. The brown seaweed known as kelp contains high levels of iodine and, in contrast to soy, has been shown to improve thyroid function.

The status of your thyroid needs to be medically evaluated, which typically involves an assessment of the thyroid hormones in your blood by a doctor knowledgeable in endocrinology. Hypothyroidism refers to a thyroid gland that is underperforming, whereas hyperthyroidism reflects an overactive thyroid.

Most processed foods suppress fat burning. These include anything that has been deep-fried, soft drinks, milk chocolate, margarine, cakes, biscuits, pies, donuts, take-out or fast-food burgers, hotdogs, sausages, and so forth. The mechanism underlying the fat-burning suppression of these foods is most likely that processed foods take fewer calories to digest than unprocessed foods. One study indicated that people burned fewer calories after eating a processed meal than after a meal composed of whole foods. Researchers first gave volunteers a cheddar cheese sandwich on whole grain bread, and then, on day two, a processed cheese sandwich on white bread. Both sandwiches had the same amount of calories. The subjects' metabolic rate was measured and revealed that 137 calories were burned after eating the sandwich made with cheddar cheese, as compared with 73 calories after eating the processed cheese sandwich. In this case, eating unprocessed food resulted in burning 43 percent more calories.

Replacing processed foods with whole foods burns more calories due to what is called the thermic effect of eating whole foods. The cheese sandwiches made with whole grain bread contained high levels of fiber, too, which lowers the surge in blood insulin levels that occurs with eating; high levels of insulin after a meal decrease fat burning. Do what you can to avoid these foods and replace them with healthy ones, such as those in the Mediterranean eating plan.

Nutrients That Reduce Fat Absorption

A number of nutrients reduce the amount of fat we absorb from what we eat. For example, drinking oolong tea—a form of green tea—with a high-fat meal significantly lowers fat absorption.[17] One study showed that the amount of total lipids and cholesterol remaining in the fecal mass of subjects increased by 52 percent after drinking 3 cups of oolong tea with each meal per day. The healthy components of green tea are called catechins, which are powerful antioxidants. Green tea contains many catechins, although epigallocatechin gallate seems to be responsible for the greatest lipid absorption effect. Epigallocatechin gallate suppresses the uptake of lipids in the small intestine and is also effective at lowering the absorption of cholesterol.

It has also been found that green tea impedes the absorption of organic pollutants, which humans can easily absorb. This leads to high levels of tissue toxicity and makes it hard to lose fat. For example, eating trans fats and oxidized and polyunsaturated vegetable oils results in increased accumulation of free radicals in our bodies. Free radicals are atoms with an odd number of electrons and are typically created when oxygen interacts with other molecules. Free radicals cause damage by reacting with the DNA inside our cells, resulting in cell death and disease. Antioxidants can prevent the negative effects of free radicals by terminating their ability to damage cells. To help the body produce enough antioxidants, a diet containing vitamins such as beta-carotene, vitamin C, and vitamin E is necessary.

Eating fruits and plants containing insect pesticides can

also allow toxins to build up in adipose cells. The accumulated toxins can be released when stimulated, which has been shown to slow fat loss and therefore may make people fat. Green tea prevents absorption of organic pollutants, so people who regularly drink green tea may experience more fat loss by reducing fat absorption in the meals they eat and by decreasing the toxic effect of organic pollutants.

Fat and Sugar in the Blood After Eating a Meal

Eating three meals per day containing 20 to 40 grams of saturated fat or 50 grams of fructose typically elevates triglyceride blood levels for up to eighteen hours. This phenomenon, postprandial lipemia, is a major risk factor for atherosclerosis and cardiovascular disease, because higher levels of fat in the blood increase inflammation and damage the lining of the arteries.

Postprandial lipemia levels vary, but they are decreased or increased by fat type, dietary intake of nutrients, and exercise. For example, consuming 30 grams or more of saturated fat typically leads to postprandial lipemia, whereas eating monounsaturated and polyunsaturated fats does not. Consuming protein, fiber, and green tea with saturated fat results in lowered postprandial lipemia, whereas drinking alcohol and smoking enhances it.[18]

One session of aerobic exercise lasting forty-five minutes resulted in significantly lower postprandial lipemia. People regularly performing aerobic exercise every week also exhibit lower postprandial lipemia. Recently, our studies have shown that twenty minutes of interval sprinting at night also reduced fat in the blood of women who ate a high-fat meal the next morning.[19]

Postprandial lipemic individuals can be inflamed for a significant proportion of the day, and this inflamed state is likely to impede fat loss. Inflammation raises the levels of insulin and cortisol, two hormones that promote fat storing. Therefore, eating meals high in saturated fat may increase belly fat stores to a greater extent than eating less saturated fat or consuming healthier fats. Those individuals who indulge in high-saturated-fat meals but consume protein, fiber, or green tea simultaneously may experience a suppressed postprandial lipemia and inflammatory response.

Eating lots of simple sugar can also cause postprandial elevations in glucose, which in turn can increase inflammation, endothelial dysfunction, and hyperinsulinemia. Endothelial dysfunction occurs when the inner lining of blood vessels functions abnormally, whereas hyperinsulinemia happens when a person has excessively high levels of insulin in their blood. Eating healthy foods such as vegetables, fruits, seeds, grains, and nuts brings about a far lower elevation of postprandial glucose.[20] Drinking one to two glasses of alcohol before eating a high-sugar meal also results in significantly lower postprandial glucose levels, and drinking a moderate amount of alcohol decreases insulin resistance for twelve to twenty-four hours. Consuming olive oil and fish oil significantly lowers postprandial blood glucose levels, and such reduction in postprandial glucose levels leads to decreased blood insulin levels. As noted previously, insulin enhances fat storage, and high blood insulin levels impede fat loss. Therefore, as discussed

with postprandial lipemia, ingesting different types of nutrients with a meal that affect postprandial glucose and insulin
could positively influence belly fat loss response.

What to Eat Before, During, and After Exercising

Digesting nutrients before, during, and after exercising influences fat burning. Eating 30 grams of fructose or glucose
one hour before a sixty-minute aerobic exercise session significantly suppressed whole body fat burning by 32 percent
(fructose) and 50 percent (glucose). Unfortunately, consuming a high-protein meal also increases blood insulin levels significantly. It is important not to eat sugar or protein
before or immediately after exercise, as these nutrients elevate blood insulin levels, which impair fat burning. Digesting low-glycemic meals before exercise also suppresses fat
oxidation, but the effect is much greater after high-glycemic
meals. Low-glycemic meals contain fewer simple sugars,
such as glucose, whereas high-glycemic meals contain lots of
glucose; consuming sugary drinks and protein snacks before
or after exercise will tend to suppress fat burning and reduce
long-term fat loss.

In contrast, other nutrients can enhance fat burning during and after exercise. For example, we have shown that
drinking green tea before interval sprinting increased fat
oxidation by over 20 percent during the hour after exercise.[21]
Another study demonstrated that having green tea before
steady-state cycle aerobic exercise resulted in a 17 percent
increase in fat oxidation during exercise.[22]

Time of Day for Optimal Belly Fat Loss with Interval Sprinting Exercise

The time of day you choose to exercise and whether or not you have eaten a meal before your session affects fat burning during exercise. Studies have shown that exercising following an overnight fast stimulates significantly greater fat burning compared with exercising soon after a meal.

One such study also investigated the effect of exercise on glucose intolerance and insulin resistance in the fasted and fed states.[23] It found that fasted training was more effective than fed training for improving glucose tolerance and insulin resistance: fasted subjects displayed greater insulin sensitivity levels than fed subjects did. The fasted subjects also significantly increased fat burning, which resulted in a much smaller weight increase in the fasted group. Thus, even though they consumed a high-calorie diet, fasted subjects gained much less weight after the six-week program. This and other studies have shown that the body burns up much more fat during and after exercise if no food is eaten beforehand. This means the best time of day to exercise in order to lose belly fat is before breakfast or your first meal.

Exercise and Appetite

Overall, the evidence indicates that engaging in exercise does not automatically increase appetite; with most people who exercise, food intake remains unchanged, and in certain circumstances, exercise may suppress appetite. It is possible that exercising may change the quality of nutrients eaten; for example, after hot, sweaty exercise, there may be a switch away from high-fat foods to fruit and water. However, this has not been examined thoroughly and is an important future research area.

Hard exercise, such as running a marathon, has been shown to induce a moderate decrease in appetite, lasting up to several hours after the session, but moderate exercise does not seem to have any effect on appetite. When people change from a sedentary lifestyle to an active one, food intake is not increased accordingly, which seems to suggest there is no biological mechanism that matches energy output to energy intake; rather, social and psychological factors may determine how much and what we eat.

The mechanisms underlying the appetite-suppressant effect incurred by hard, vigorous exercise are unknown, but increased body temperature may inhibit food intake; people in cold climates normally eat more than those in temperate or warm regions. Recent research has also found that a number of gut peptides change after exercise and may inhibit food intake by suppressing signals from the GI tract to the brain.[24] Gut peptides are involved in the control of food intake and can make us feel full or hungry. Other studies have shown that satiety hormones released from the brain during hard exercise also suppress appetite, and that elevated blood lactate levels blunt appetite by affecting appetite centers in the brain.[25] In contrast, however, other studies have shown that cold-water workouts increase appetite, with individuals who exercise in cool water eating more afterward.[26] The effect of interval sprinting on appetite has not been examined and is an important area for future research, but we already know that blood levels of lactate rise during interval sprinting.

Successful fat loss involves lifestyle changes, *not* short-term starvation. The components of healthy living—healthy eating, exercise, limiting stress, and quality sleep—all interact to influence our body composition and health. The Mediterranean eating plan is ideal for people in the Western industrialized world, as it requires minimal preparation and does not involve counting calories.

*

This chapter has emphasized what we should be eating. The ideal way to eat for optimum health includes:

- Avoid processed foods with added sugar.

- Consume those saturated fats that are good for health (coconut, avocado), while eliminating those that are bad for health.

- Consume those polyunsaturated and monounsaturated oils that are good for health (olive oil, fish oil), while eliminating those that are bad for health, such as vegetable oils.

- Eat plants full of fiber (apples, coconut, strawberries).

- Reduce or eliminate animal protein, as too much is bad for health, and replace it with beneficial plant proteins.

- Follow the Mediterranean eating plan, as it is the only diet that has been documented to help people lose fat and keep it off.

The right kind of exercise, combined with a healthy, nutritious eating program, is a step in the right direction to losing belly fat and keeping it off. But these are not the only factors that lead to fat gain. Our busy modern lives leave us more stressed and less rested, two factors that prompt our bodies to put on dangerous belly fat. Chapter 5 looks at ways of managing your stress level and how to get enough sleep to gain the full benefit from your belly fat reduction program.

Chapter 5
Reducing Daily Stress and Enhancing Sleep Quality

Stress is a process that happens when people respond to environmental and psychological stressors that generate challenge or danger. Stress stimulates the "fight or flight" center in the brain, which bring about the release of stress hormones such as catecholamines and cortisol. The catecholamines increase our breathing rate to provide more oxygen to muscles, elevate heart rate and blood pressure, and mobilize fat into the blood for extra energy. Muscles also can become tense, and people under stress often find that their mouths become dry and they begin sweating. In addition, cortisol, another stress hormone, helps store fat and releases sugar into the blood.

The stress response is not always generated by the situation alone—the anticipation of a potential stressor can also have a significant impact on how stress affects an individual. A moderate amount of stress can add interest to daily life and can help us adapt to change, but too much stress has been shown to contribute to a range of health problems, such as heart attack, gastrointestinal problems, hypertension, stroke, diabetes, cancer, tuberculosis, insomnia, pneumonia, influenza, headaches, and an increase in belly fat.

There are three main types of stressors: cataclysmic stress, personal stress, and daily stress. A cataclysmic stressor occurs infrequently but is typically life changing. For example, major floods, abnormally cold weather, tornadoes, and plane and train crashes greatly disrupt people's lives and can typically bring about a significant stress response. Personal stressors are usually infrequent but can be equally stressful: the death of a loved one or going through a painful divorce has been shown to generate stress. Daily stressors involve the frustrations that many of us experience, such as commuting in busy traffic, dealing with incompetent coworkers, having too much to do in too little time, and so forth. These stressors can occur frequently throughout the day and have the ability to constantly generate a stress response.

The Effect of Stress on Belly Fat

The major stress hormone that leads to increased deposits of belly fat is cortisol; at high levels in the circulation, this chemical messenger tells the liver to release sugar into the blood, bringing about an increase in blood insulin levels. Constant high levels of cortisol and insulin in the blood encourage fat accumulation and an increase in belly fat.

There is a link among stress, cortisol, and appetite, as

Measuring your daily stress

The amount of daily stress in your life can be assessed in the test below. If you score more than 20 points, you have high levels of stress and need to take action to reduce your daily stress levels. Answer the six questions using a score of 1 to 4 for each question, and then add up your total.

1 = Not at all   2 = Sometimes

3 = Fairly regularly   4 = All the time

1. I worry about personal problems in my life every day

2. My personal problems interfere with my job and relationships

3. I constantly feel that things in my life are out of control

4. I feel the stress in my life affects my health

5. I find the stress in my life disrupts my sleep

6. I often feel anxious and irritable during the day

TOTAL

Interpreting your score:

6 to 9 points: low levels of daily stress

10 to 12 points: moderately low levels of daily stress

13 to 18 points: moderately high levels of daily stress

19 to 24 points: high levels of daily stress

studies have shown that injecting people with cortisol increased their appetite and their craving for sugar. Young women who secreted more cortisol while stressed also ate more sugar and fat afterward. Cortisol may influence appetite by binding to receptors in the hypothalamus, a part of the brain that controls appetite. This can cause people to consume more junk food, which contains large amounts of fat and sugar. Cortisol also regulates other chemicals that control appetite. For example, stress hormones such as corticotropin-releasing factor and neuropeptide Y have been shown to stimulate appetite. Exposure to stressors also elevates inflammation levels, which have been implicated in the development of obesity.

How to Cope with Stress

There are a number of ways to cope with stress, including taking direct action against and seeking information about the stressor, inhibiting stressful actions, and employing general stress-management habits. For example, if a person's job is his or her main source of stress, then the best solution would be to find another job. Unfortunately, for most people, this is not practical, so they have to find a way of coping with the stress generated by their jobs. If driving in morning traffic is stressful, then a way to cope might be to get information about traffic flow during different times of the day, to provide options for decreasing the stressful effects of traffic.

Another coping mechanism is to stop fighting the stressor and accept it; this is called inhibiting the stressor. It does not get rid of the stressor but saves the energy and effort required for coping with it. For example, rather than getting angry every time you find yourself mired in morning traffic, you could accept that city roads will always be busy during rush hour and play music to help you relax rather than get upset.

Finally, if a stressor cannot be removed or inhibited, stress management offers a number of strategies and techniques to reduce or stop the deleterious effects of exposure to daily stressors. Read on and learn how to use stress-management skills such as controlled breathing, muscle relaxation, and imagery to avoid becoming agitated.

Stress Management

Stress management typically involves managing stressors wherever possible, modifying your perception of stressful situations, developing stress-resistance resources, controlling stress reactions, controlled breathing, muscle relaxation, and imagery. More information on these strategies can be found in *Minding the Body, Mending the Mind* by Joan Borysenko.[1] From a belly fat perspective, the most important strategies include the use of exercise and the development of controlled breathing, muscle relaxation, imagery, and time-management skills to cope with stress.

CONTROLLED BREATHING

Controlled breathing is a stress-management technique that concentrates on slowing and optimizing your breathing. Rapid breathing quickly produces a number of unwanted physiological responses, such as an elevated heart rate and feelings of dizziness.

A warm, darkened, carpeted room is recommended when learning how to control your breathing and muscle tension. You should lie on your back with your arms by your side; you can lie on the floor or a firm bed. Make sure that your clothing is not tight or uncomfortable. Finally, make sure you do not have any injuries that cause discomfort when lying in this position. Now follow the steps listed below.

1. Close your eyes and focus your thoughts on your breathing.

2. Slow your breathing and take deep, even breaths. Focus all your thoughts on the air as it enters your nasal passage and progresses deep into your lungs. If extraneous thoughts enter your mind, push them aside and refocus all your attention on your breathing.

3. Now concentrate on your breathing cue word: *relax*. As you say the word in your mind, breathe in on the *re* and out on the *lax*. One cycle should take about 5 seconds—2.5 seconds breathing in, and 2.5 seconds breathing out—which equates to twelve breathing cycles per minute. Practice using this cue for three breathing cycles. Remember, slowly breathe in on the *re* and slowly breathe out on the *lax*.

4. If thoughts enter your mind or noises come to your attention, push them aside and refocus all your concentration on your breathing.

5. As you practice the muscle relaxation technique in the next section, try to monitor and control your breathing throughout the session using your cue word: *relax*.

MUSCLE RELAXATION

Muscle relaxation is a technique that systematically releases all the tension in your skeletal muscles. As with the controlled breathing technique, you should lie on your back with your arms by your side in a warm, darkened room. Try to wear comfortable, nonrestrictive clothing. Follow the instructions below to learn how muscle relaxation is performed for the whole body.

1. Lie on your back on a carpeted floor or on a firm bed. Support your head with a small cushion. Allow your legs and arms to stretch out. If you suffer from lower back problems, place a rolled-up blanket under your knees.

2. To begin, complete a body tension check by monitoring all your muscle groups for excessive muscle tension. Close your eyes and scan the muscles in your body from your head to your feet. Try to sense which of your muscles are tense. Don't forget about your breathing; it should be slow and even.

3. Now start muscle relaxation: tense your fist by curling your fingers as tight as you can for fifteen seconds. Hold the tension and focus on it; then release by relaxing your hands and letting your fingers slowly uncurl.

Notice the warm, tingling sensation of relaxed muscles, compared with the earlier feeling of tension.

4. Next, focus on your biceps: Create tension in these upper-arm muscles for fifteen seconds by lifting both hands to the shoulders and tightening the biceps. Try to keep your hands relaxed. Now release the tension in your biceps by relaxing them and letting your arms slowly return to your sides.

5. Now tense your neck muscles by contracting and pushing the back of your neck into the pillow for fifteen seconds. Hold the tension, focus on it, and then release it by relaxing your neck.

6. Tense your facial muscles by frowning and gritting your teeth for fifteen seconds. Hold the tension, focus on it, and then release it by relaxing.

7. Now contract your abdominal muscles by tensing and pulling in your stomach for fifteen seconds. Hold the tension, focus on it, and then release it by relaxing.

8. Next, continue with your thighs and buttocks. Tense these muscles tightly for fifteen seconds and then release the tension.

9. Don't forget to focus on your breathing by using your cue word, *relax*. Take a deep breath on the *re,* hold your breath, and then release it on the *lax*.

10. Finish by tensing your lower legs. Keep your eyes closed and contract your feet and lower legs by pushing them

into the carpet or bed. Hold the tension for fifteen seconds and then relax. By now you should feel your body getting warm and heavy.

11. Once you have completed the exercise, remain lying down for a while. You may go to sleep, so if you have other things to do, set an alarm clock before you begin.

IMAGERY RELAXATION

Much stress is caused by thinking about negative situations. For some people, relaxing muscles may not be enough, and they must also relax their minds by blocking stressful thoughts and trying to stop worrying. Relaxation imagery involves imagining a relaxing scene by using sight, sound, smell, and touch, which distracts a stressed person from worrying.

Choose a relaxing image that you most associate with calmness, peace, tranquility, serenity, and harmony. It might be a real-life scenario, such as walking through the countryside, or a fantasy image, such as drifting along with the clouds. Try to involve all your senses in your imagery, so think about what you can see, hear, touch, and smell. The two practice images described in the instructions below involve clouds and a warm house in winter. Try these images and then develop your own.

When practicing relaxation imagery, a warm, darkened, carpeted room is recommended. You should lie on your back with your arms by your side. Make sure your clothing is not tight or uncomfortable. Also make sure you do not have any injuries that cause you discomfort when lying in this position.

Now close your eyes and create the following scene in your mind. You are on a warm, white beach. You are the only person there, the water is calm and green, and the sky is a vivid blue. Focus on the sky. In your mind's eye, you see nothing but blue. Now focus on the green and turquoise colors of the sea. Focus on the smell of the ocean; let the fresh smell of the sea flood your mind. You can feel a gentle sea breeze against your face. Next, focus on the sky, where you can see a small white cloud descending slowly to the beach. The cloud becomes larger until it finally settles under you. You are lying on top of this small cloud. It gently lifts you into the air, and you see the beach becoming smaller and smaller. Your body is becoming lighter and lighter. You feel warm, secure, and relaxed.

Now the cloud descends, and your body is feeling more relaxed. As the cloud touches the beach, you feel warm, heavy, and relaxed. Focus on your breathing. Use your cue word—*relax*—for two breathing cycles. At the end of the second cycle, open your eyes. You should feel energized and ready for action.

Now for your second imagery relaxation exercise: picture a warm house in the middle of winter. With your eyes closed, think about the home: Is it a country house or a town house? Is it modern or old? What sort of houseplants are there? Can you hear the cold wind outside? Can you feel the warmth inside the house? Perhaps you can smell the aroma of your favorite food drifting from the kitchen. Move through each room of the house, concentrating on what you can see, hear, smell, and feel before going on to the next image. Once you have spent a short time exploring, you should know your house so well that you could describe it to someone else.

*

Note that when you use relaxation imagery techniques, it is not the same as visualizing with your eyes open. When visualizing with your eyes open, you get a sharp, focused picture that remains steady. In contrast, mental images tend to be more fluid—more like ideas of what something looks like rather than a reproduction of reality.

RELAXATION ON THE GO

If stress symptoms seize you in the workplace, following some of the strategies below may help you manage your daily work stressors. At some point during the workday, take a five-minute break when you can:

- sit down and have a healthy snack, such as a piece of fruit;

- remove yourself from your working environment by going outside and walking around;

- find a quiet place and practice the breathing, muscle relaxation, and imagery techniques;

- withdraw to somewhere quiet, close your eyes, and allow your body to rest; or

- if you are working from home, put on a favorite piece of music. Sit or lie down with your eyes closed and listen for a while.

TIME MANAGEMENT

Many of the daily hassles that cause us stress on a regular basis are caused by poor time management. Many people are simply not well organized, and trying to do too much in an unplanned fashion can generate the stress response. Characteristics of efficient time management include developing a long-term plan, prioritizing and planning ahead, and using a yearly planner. Planning on a weekly basis involves filling in a weekly planner, using time slots wisely, being flexible, being realistic, and seeking help. Common "time thieves" are procrastinating, wasting time on irrelevant tasks, failing to start a task, drifting off, being a perfectionist, and putting tasks into the too-hard basket. Some easy-to-follow time-management tips include completing small tasks straightaway, breaking tasks into small, manageable units, and developing a goal-setting plan.

Goals are really useful for getting things done. Guidelines for effective goal setting include:

- Set specific, measurable goals.

- Set difficult but realistic goals.

- Set short-range goals.

- Set goals based on performance rather than outcomes.

• Set positive goals, not negative ones.

• Identify target dates.

• Record your goals in a yearly planner.

• Evaluate your goals.

An example of short-term goal setting is to complete three weekly twenty-minute interval sprinting sessions, eat a piece of fruit each day, and practice muscle relaxation nightly for one week. At the end of the week the completion success of these goals should be evaluated. For example, if practicing muscle relaxation every night was too demanding, then try three times per week.

Common obstacles that prevent people from meeting their goals include setting too many goals, making goals too general, setting unrealistic goals, and setting outcome-oriented goals. A goal-setting system allows you to assess your needs, set yourself long- and short-term goals, and evaluate your progress and adjust your goals weekly.

How to Use the Breathing, Muscle Relaxation, Imagery Relaxation, and Time-Management Techniques

You should try all these basic stress-management techniques to see which ones work best for you. Whatever you decide, an effective way of learning and performing the relaxation techniques is to make a tape or a script. Simply read out loud and record the scripts in each of the exercises above on a cassette player or using your phone's Record function, and then practice the skills by playing and listening to the recording.

Ideally, you should try relaxing daily or at least three times per week. As you develop these relaxation skills, the protocols may be shortened and transferred to more realistic settings, which is called differential relaxation, though this may take weeks. Progression of differential relaxation could be: relaxing in a chair; relaxing in a car or train; relaxing during stressful situations during the day. Learning to monitor and control anxiety and tension can be achieved through a sound goal-setting system and well-structured stress-management skill sessions.

EXERCISE AND STRESS REDUCTION

The autonomic, cardiac, and vascular changes that occur following participation in regular aerobic exercise are well documented. For example, low resting heart rate—bradycardia—typically occurs with regular aerobic exercise such as running. Resting heart rates of trained runners are often less than 50 beats per minute. Heart rate during an exercise session is also decreased after training.

These changes have prompted researchers to speculate that because regular aerobic exercise makes the body more efficient at handling exercise stress, then at the same time it will also produce a more efficient response to psychological stress. There is mixed evidence, however, to suggest that frequent physical activity may decrease the physiological response to stress in healthy individuals. The major finding appears to be that aerobic fitness is associated with slightly better heart-rate recovery from stress.[2]

A decrease in the stress response has been found in those few studies that have examined men and women at cardiovascular risk, such as people whose parents suffered from hypertension or who have hypertension themselves, and we know that the blunted skeletal muscle blood flow and increased blood pressure response to stress commonly found in the overweight and viscerally obese can be normalized with regular exercise.

These results have been derived mainly from studies using steady-state aerobic exercise such as cycling, jogging, and swimming, but the effects of other types of exercise, such as interval sprinting, on the stress response are poorly explored. We have shown that one session of interval sprinting, compared with one of steady-state exercise, produced a significantly greater impact on the autonomic nervous system, as assessed by heart rate and blood levels of catecholamine levels.[3] Regular interval sprinting training also resulted in a significant change in resting cardiovascular and autonomic function.[4]

Given that interval sprinting induces a significant acute cardiovascular response, it is possible that interval sprinting training may also produce greater adaptations to the stress response. Recently, we examined the effect of interval sprinting on the stress response. We found that twelve weeks of sprinting produced significant differences in cardiovascular and autonomic response during exposure to a laboratory stressor.[5] Specifically, men who performed twelve weeks of interval sprinting experienced a significant reduction in heart rate during a challenging computer task. Exercisers, compared with a group of volunteers, also showed decreased stiffness of their large arteries and increased muscle blood flow during stress.

There are a number of other ways to use exercise to help relieve the stress in our lives. As mentioned earlier, regular involvement in physical activity such as interval sprinting causes the body to adapt to both exercise and psychological stress. We know that exercisers have significantly less incidence of cardiovascular disease and stroke, but how much of this effect is due to a reduced stress response is unknown. Another way of using exercise to buffer the stress response is to use it as a "time-out": after a busy morning at work, taking a fifty-minute jog around a pleasant park at lunchtime may simply distract an individual from the stress of work. Similarly, participating in twenty minutes of interval sprinting while listening to invigorating music may also direct people's thoughts away from daily stressors. However, more research on the stress-reducing capacity of interval sprinting is needed.

Sleep It Off

Most human behaviors have an obvious purpose. For example, we eat to provide energy for the body and drink water to supply fluid in and around the cells. Up to 30 percent of a person's life may be spent in sleep; however, the physiological function of sleep is unknown. The two main hypotheses to explain why we have to sleep are restoration and protection. The restoration hypothesis suggests that we sleep to restore the energy depletion that occurred during the previous day. However, approximately the same amount of energy is expended while sitting and sleeping. Moreover, bedridden people sleep more than healthy people. The protective hypothesis suggests that our nervous system carries hardwired behavioral patterns; because we lack adequate night sensors, it is safer to sleep at night. Whatever the reason for sleeping, it is known that lack of sleep or poor-quality, nonrefreshing sleep has an adverse effect on health; after the common cold, sleep problems are the second-biggest health complaint, and there are over fifty identified sleep disorders.

People experiencing regular sleep disruption typically possess greater body and belly fat than people who sleep well. Sleep-deprived people also face greater difficulty losing fat after a diet or exercise intervention. Differences in the number of hours of sleep also influence body composition, as it has been shown that people who sleep less tend to be overweight.[6] Disrupted sleep may change the balance between satiety hormones that control hunger, as sleeping five hours per night results in greater ghrelin and less leptin levels compared with sleeping eight hours. Leptin, a hormone secreted by fat cells, tells the brain that we have had enough to eat, while ghrelin, secreted from the lining of the gut, transmits the message "I'm hungry!" Thus, sleep deprivation affects body fat accumulation because it makes us hungrier. Increased resting cortisol levels have also been found in people who experience lack of sleep. As a result, sleeping well is very important for helping the body spend longer in fat-burning mode than in fat-storing mode.

The Effect of Sleep on Health

Together with healthy eating, exercise, and stress management, sleep is now acknowledged as one of the four pillars of a healthy lifestyle. Poor-quality sleep can have a major effect on people's emotional state and their ability to concentrate and remember. Also, sleep disorders such as obstructive sleep apnea contribute to hypertension development, type 2 diabetes, and cardiovascular disease. Poor-quality sleep also causes decreased productivity and an increase in workplace and driving accidents. The US Centers for Disease Control and Prevention have estimated that sleep disorders cost society over $18 billion per year.

There are many sleep disorders, but the major ones in adults are insomnia, narcolepsy, and sleep apnea. Insomnia is characterized by difficulty falling asleep, waking up frequently, waking up too early, and nonrefreshing sleep. In sleep apnea, a person's breathing pauses during sleep. Apnea sufferers, often unaware of their problem, cope with daytime sleepiness and fatigue, snore regularly, and their throat muscle, and tongue, relax too much when sleeping.

Obese people tend to develop sleep apnea more than people of normal weight do, and it is more common in men and in older individuals. Sleep apnea patients typically have low blood-oxygen levels and increased stress hormone levels; abnormally high blood pressure; a greater incidence of heart attack, stroke, heart failure, and irregular heartbeats;

Measuring the quality of your sleep

The quality of your sleep can be assessed by using the test below. Answer the six questions, using a score of 1 to 4 for each question, and then add up your total. If you score less than 4 points, then you have poor-quality sleep and need to take action to improve your sleep.

1 = Not at all   2 = Sometimes

3 = Fairly regularly   4 = All the time

1. I have difficulty falling asleep within fifteen minutes

2. I wake up in the middle of the night or early morning

3. I constantly feel too hot or too cold in bed

4. I wake up too early and can't get back to sleep

5. I regularly have bad dreams

6. On waking, I feel tired and do not feel refreshed

TOTAL

Interpreting your score:

6 to 9 points: good-quality sleep

10 to 12 points: moderately good-quality sleep

13 to 18 points: moderately poor-quality sleep

19 to 24 points: very poor-quality sleep

and increased work-related or driving accidents. The treatment for sleep apnea involves positive airway pressure, mouthpieces, sleeping on one's side, oxygen, practicing wind instruments such as flute and oboe, surgery, and lifestyle changes. Positive airway pressure therapy involves using a machine to bring about easier breathing during sleep. Sleep apnea treatment can also involve using a mouthpiece device to keep your airway open. Some people undergo a surgical procedure to change their nose, mouth, or throat structure.

The Effect of Sleep on Belly Fat

A study published in the journal *Sleep* found that sleep duration was related to increases in belly fat.[7] Results showed that people sleeping less than five hours a night gained more belly fat over five years, compared with people sleeping over six hours a night. Short sleepers experienced a 32 percent gain in belly fat, compared with a 13 percent gain for people who slept six or seven hours each night. Individuals who slept at least eight hours a night showed a 22 percent increase in belly fat for both men and women over the five-year period. Short and long sleepers found it more difficult to fall asleep, woke more often during the night, woke up early in the morning and could not get back to sleep, and suffered from fatigue during the day compared to those who slept six to seven hours.

Another study, carried out by the National Sleep Foundation in 2003, found that older men and women who slept poorly were more likely to develop type 2 diabetes. There was a higher incidence of sleep problems in older adults who were obese or overweight, though about half of older adults exercised three or more times per week. The more that older people exercised, the less likely they were to report poor-quality sleep.

Sleep Onset

Change in body temperature directly affects sleep onset. Body core temperature refers to the temperature in organs and tissue deep inside the body, such as the brain and the spinal cord, whereas skin temperature is the temperature of the extremities of the body, such as the hands and feet. When body core temperature increases, people tend to be more active and awake. In contrast, when body core temperature drops, they become sleepy.

A hormone called melatonin is produced by the brain's pineal gland at night and initiates the sleep cycle by lowering body core temperature. Melatonin levels are reduced by aging, by exposure to bright light, and by lack of sleep. Consequently, older adults, those exposed to bright light, and shift workers or those who do not enjoy adequate sleep are likely to have reduced melatonin and an impaired ability to sleep well.

Studies have shown that after taking acetaminophen or aspirin right before sleep, people fall asleep more quickly. This effect is attributed to these drugs' ability to lower the body's core temperature. A research group at the University of Pittsburgh also showed that when the front of insomniacs' heads were cooled by a special cooling cap, they slept as well as normal sleepers. As discussed below, hot, sweaty exercise may enhance the onset and quality of sleep by lowering core temperature.

Strategies for increasing sleep quality include:

- Avoid vigorous exercise directly before bedtime. Leave at least two hours between aerobic exercise and going to bed.

- Gently stretching for one to two minutes before bed may help you relax.

- Eat your evening meal at least one hour before bed, but don't go to bed hungry, as being hungry may keep you awake.

- Listen to the radio (not TV) as you lie in bed with your eyes closed. This is an effective way of falling asleep.

- Ensure you have a comfortable, good-quality bed.

- Have a warm (not hot) bath last thing at night.

- Drink warm herbal tea a half hour before bedtime. Chamomile is particularly relaxing.

- Avoid alcohol, caffeine, and nicotine for at least five hours before bed. By not drinking late you can avoid waking up in the middle of the night with the urge to urinate.

- Establish a steady bedtime routine with a regular time to go to bed and to rise.

- Try not to discuss work or domestic problems in bed. Treat your bed as your sanctuary where work issues are not allowed. Set a "worry-time" before sleeping, after which you can put worrisome thoughts out of your mind.

Exercise and Sleep

Exercise has an important role to play in enhancing the quality of sleep. Hot, sweaty aerobic exercise in the late afternoon has been shown to result in better sleep. Sauna baths (thermal therapy) have also been shown to improve sleep quality if taken in the late afternoon. The exercise mechanism may be the same as that in thermal therapy. During hot, sweaty exercise, body core temperature increases, but after exercise has stopped, body core temperature starts to fall. As mentioned previously, when body core temperature goes down, people become sleepy. Thus, exercise may increase sleep quality by influencing sleep centers in the brain such as the hypothalamus and sleep hormones such as melatonin. Exercise in the morning, however, does not appear to affect sleep onset or quality. There are a number of things to consider when using exercise to increase the quality of your sleep:

- Exercise in the late afternoon.

- Use vigorous aerobic exercise that induces sweating.

- Participating in resistance exercise does not appear to improve sleep quality.

- The effect of interval sprinting on sleep quality is unknown.

*

It's clear that high levels of stress and not enough sleep can severely affect our health, and that we can improve our health by improving stress management and poor-quality sleep. The key points to keep in mind are:

- People who have high levels of daily stress and who sleep poorly tend to have higher levels of cortisol in their blood and typically acquire more belly fat.

- There are a number of dietary and behavioral strategies you can use to reduce the effects of stress and to enhance sleep quality.

- Relaxation techniques and interval sprint training can help you cope with stress, while moderately vigorous aerobic exercise in the late afternoon is more effective than less vigorous exercise for sleep enhancement.

Chapter 6

A Six-Week Belly Fat Loss Program

As has been discussed previously, many of the key health benefits of interval sprinting emerge after six weeks. Just one hour of interval sprinting each week for six weeks can significantly decrease belly fat, as measured by waist circumference and insulin resistance. Interval sprinting has also been shown to significantly increase leg and abdominal muscle mass and aerobic fitness. We consider interval sprinting one of the four pillars of health, along with healthy eating, controlling the effect of daily stress, and ensuring good-quality sleep. It is clear that making changes in these other areas will further enhance the health benefits of interval sprinting. This chapter contains a six-week lifestyle program for anyone who requires change in each of those four areas. The goals for each component are listed, together with examples of a weekly program.

To begin the program, first complete the self-tests that assess your fitness levels (appendixes A and B, pages 183 and 185) and add them to those you completed earlier for your body composition (appendix E, page 191), your diet (chapter 4), your amount of daily stress (chapter 5), and your sleep quality (chapter 5). It's a good idea to photocopy these pages so that you can continue to assess your performance as the program progresses. Keeping records will help you to adjust the program according to your individual assessment, your personal preferences, and time availability.

Developing an Interval Sprinting Program

Choose a form of exercise, such as cycling or sprint skipping, from those described in chapter 3. If you settle on the stationary bike, select a pedalling rate and resistance to help determine your exercise intensity. Other forms of interval sprinting, such as swimming, may involve only determining the rate. Decide how many times per week you want to sprint, at what intensity, and for how long each session.

It is important to perform interval sprinting with the correct technique and at the optimal intensity. Details on developing the best interval sprinting program for your level of fitness and health are described in chapter 3.

Interval Sprinting Guidelines

- Have your health checked before undertaking interval sprinting.

- Determine the mode, rate, and exercise intensity preferable for you.

- Gradually increase the length and intensity of your training during the first two weeks.

Examples of light, moderate, and hard interval sprinting programs that can be performed in the morning, at lunchtime, and in the evening are described in chapter 3.

Adding an Interval Sprinting Exercise Program for the Upper Body

A lower- and upper-body interval sprinting protocol on alternate days is likely to result in a better total body workout than just a lower-body program. For example, a session of rowing, boxing, or rope skipping as a combination or individually for twenty minutes is likely to bring extra health benefits. Of course, if you can do only sixty minutes of exercise a week, then the three twenty-minute sessions on the stationary bike are optimal. This would still add up to only one hour of interval sprinting per week, plus twenty-four minutes of warm-up and cool-down. An example of a lower- and upper-body interval sprinting program at a light intensity is described in table 10.

	Before sprinting	Time of day: 6:00 a.m. to 8:00 a.m.	Pedal rate and resistance	Information recorded
Monday	Drink water or green tea	20 minutes LifeSprints on the bike	90 rpm at 0.5 kg, with 50 rpm recovery	Weight and fat, exercise heart rate, and RPE
Tuesday	Drink water or green tea	20 minutes rowing, skipping, or boxing	See page 91	Exercise heart rate and RPE
Wednesday	Drink water or green tea	20 minutes LifeSprints on the bike	90 rpm at 0.5 kg, with 50 rpm recovery	Exercise heart rate and RPE
Thursday	Drink water or green tea	20 minutes rowing, skipping, or boxing	See page 94	Exercise heart rate and RPE
Friday	Drink water or green tea	20 minutes LifeSprints on the bike	90 rpm at 0.5 kg, with 50 rpm recovery	Exercise heart rate and RPE
Saturday	Rest day			
Sunday	Drink water or green tea	20 minutes rowing, skipping, or boxing	See page 96	Exercise heart rate and RPE

Table 10. Example of lower- and upper-body interval sprinting program at light intensity

Adopting the Mediterranean Eating Plan

To gain the best results from your interval training program, you should make an assessment of your current diet by completing the diet assessment in chapter 4 (page 106) or by using a free online dietary analysis program like Nutridiary (www.nutridiary.com).

If you have an unhealthy diet, follow the Mediterranean plan for six weeks, as outlined in chapter 4. Most people will not need to count calories on this diet. After three weeks, you should feel more energetic and less tired. The recipes for Monday's and Tuesday's meals are included in chapter 4; please consult the endnotes for recipes for the week's remaining meals.

Controlling Daily Stress

As well as an interval sprinting and healthy eating program, it's important to limit the amount of stress in your life for optimum belly fat loss. As discussed in chapter 5, individuals exposed to stressors may increase their belly fat stores due to elevated cortisol and insulin levels.

Regular exercise, breathing, muscle relaxation, imagery, and time-management skills are likely to be helpful in reducing the negative effects of daily stressors. Poor-quality sleep also results in elevated cortisol levels and increased belly fat; thus stress-management techniques and sleep-quality-enhancement strategies need to be implemented.

	Breakfast	Lunch	Dinner
Monday	Scrambled egg on toast; green or black tea, or water; 1 piece of whole fruit	Curried vegetables (recipe p. 128); green or black tea, or water; mixed fruit	Roasted salmon and asparagus; wine*; dark chocolate; fruit, nuts
Tuesday	Fruit salad with yogurt; green or black tea, or water	Spicy burrito (recipe p. 129); green or black tea, or water; mixed fruit	Lemon caper chicken with couscous; wine; fruit
Wednesday	Cereal with fruit; green or black tea, or water	Fish tacos with avocado and salsa;[1] green or black tea, or water; mixed fruit	Shrimp and vegetable quinoa fried rice;[6] wine; fruit, nuts
Thursday	Scrambled egg on toast; green or black tea, or water; 1 piece of whole fruit	Tahini tuna salad;[2] green or black tea, or water; mixed fruit	Tandoori chicken with fresh vegetables and rice;[7] wine; fruit
Friday	Fruit salad with yogurt; green or black tea, or water	Garden vegetable wrap;[3] green or black tea, or water; mixed fruit	Grilled halibut with avocado sauce;[8] wine; fruit, nuts
Saturday	Cereal with fruit; green or black tea, or water	Black bean salad;[4] green or black tea, or water; mixed fruit	Steak stir-fry with vegetables;[9] red wine; dark chocolate; fruit
Sunday	Fruit salad with yogurt; green or black tea, or water	Satay chicken with steamed vegetables;[5] green or black tea, or water; mixed fruit	Cod poached in tomato sauce with spinach, capers and pine nuts;[10] wine; fruit, nuts

Table 11. Sample week of mediterranean eating plan

Limit is 1 glass for women and 2 for men

Below is an example of a practice schedule for stress-management strategies, for implementing alongside interval sprinting and healthy eating:

Monday	20 minutes of muscle relaxation and breathing
Tuesday	10 minutes of imagery
Wednesday	20 minutes of muscle relaxation and breathing
Thursday	10 minutes of imagery
Friday	20 minutes of muscle relaxation and breathing
Saturday	
Sunday	

Table 12. Stress-management practice schedule

Enhancing Quality of Sleep

If, after completing your sleep-quality assessment in chapter 5 (page 167), you find that your sleep needs improvement, you can work your way through the suggested techniques and tips to see which ones work best for you. For example, you could set a goal of creating a presleep routine, perhaps aiming to drink a cup of herbal tea and do ten minutes of relaxation using the imagery technique every night.

Consuming the Appropriate Nutrients Before and After Interval Sprinting

As discussed in chapter 4 (page 143), digesting nutrients before, during, and after interval sprinting affects fat burning. Consuming sugary drinks and eating protein snacks before exercise will impede fat burning and reduce long-term fat loss, while other nutrients can enhance fat burning after and during exercise. Drinking green tea before exercise significantly increases fat burning during the hour after a session of interval sprinting.

Exercising in the morning, before eating, is the ideal time to burn more fat during exercise and to put the body into fat-burning mode. Drink water or good-quality green tea before, during, and after exercise, but try to refrain from eating for at least forty-five minutes after exercise. If you can exercise only during your lunch hour, the best strategy would be to not eat anything for three hours before exercising.

*

The four pillars of a healthy lifestyle have now been described, and suggested programs for interval sprinting, healthy eating, stress management, and sleep quality have been outlined. An example of a weekly program involving these four critical behaviors is: (1) twenty minutes of bike interval sprinting, three times per week; (2) Mediterranean eating every day; (3) daily stress-management technique practice; and (4) the use of sleep-quality-enhancement strategies every night.

Try it for six weeks, recording your results at the same time each week, and discover the difference that just one hour of interval training a week can make.

Monitoring Progress

As described in chapter 3, to monitor your progress, you need to record a certain amount of information. This information could include the following:

- heart-rate response during exercise;

- heart-rate response during the four-minute cool-down;

- pedal rate during bike exercise;

- pedal resistance during bike exercise;

- rating of perceived exertion (RPE) during exercise;

- weight and/or body fat change;

- waist circumference change;

- abdominal width change;

- waist skinfold site change;

- midthigh circumference change;

- lower leg circumference change;

- diet assessment;

- daily stress-level assessment; and

- quality-of-sleep assessment.

What to Expect

We and other research groups have shown that because interval sprinting imposes greater loads on all three muscle fiber types (slow, intermediate, and fast-twitch), its impact on total fat and belly fat, aerobic fitness, insulin resistance, and muscle mass is both greater and quicker than that of other forms of exercise.[11] As the average person does not have the equipment or expertise to directly measure these health changes, indirect and simple measures can be utilized. We have shown that many of these positive changes can occur after six weeks—just eighteen sessions—of properly performed interval sprinting on a stationary bike.

Over the last ten years, we have witnessed a consistent increase in the amount of studies examining different aspects of interval sprinting in research labs in the United States, Europe, Australia, and Asia. The results have been impressive and consistent. We have no doubt that, for reducing belly fat and decreasing insulin resistance, interval sprinting is the premier form of exercise. Given that it produces these effects with at least half the exercise time, it is ideal for those of us with busy lives.

We have given you a substantial amount of information in this book, but it's up to you how you use it: for some, the information on how to do interval sprinting may be enough; for others, changing their whole lifestyle may be appealing.

We believe that embarking on an interval sprinting program will significantly enhance your quality of life and may even prevent or decrease the effect of a number of lifestyle-related diseases.

And it takes only six weeks.

Appendix A
The Cooper Twelve-Minute Walk/Run Fitness Test

This twelve-minute fitness test is a convenient way to assess aerobic fitness. The test assumes that there is a reasonable relationship between the distance a person can run or walk in twelve minutes and his or her maximum aerobic fitness. The aerobic values achieved through this easy field test can be compared with those of people of the same age and gender. Test results, however, are affected by motivational factors; thus, being less or more motivated to run or walk could influence test results.

To perform the Cooper Twelve-Minute Walk/Run Fitness Test, you have to run or walk as far as you can in twelve minutes. It is usually completed on a running track, and a stopwatch is required to make sure that you walk/run for twelve minutes exactly. This test can be demanding, so make sure you have a physician's clearance.

First, warm up for eight to ten minutes, and then run or walk as far as you can in twelve minutes. After you have completed the test, compare your results with the norms below.

Age	Excellent	Above Average	Average	Below Average	Poor
Males 20 to 29	Greater than 1.7 miles	1.5 to 1.7 miles	1.4 to 1.5 miles	1.0 to 1.4 miles	Less than 1.0 mile
Males 30 to 39	Greater than 1.7 miles	1.4 to 1.7 miles	1.2 to 1.4 miles	0.9 to 1.2 miles	Less than 0.9 mile
Males 40 to 49	Greater than 1.6 miles	1.3 to 1.6 miles	1.1 to 1.3 miles	0.9 to 1.1 miles	Less than 0.9 mile
Males 50 and older	Greater than 1.5 miles	1.2 to 1.5 miles	1.0 to 1.2 miles	0.8 to 1.0 miles	Less than 0.8 mile
Females 20 to 29	Greater than 1.7 miles	1.4 to 1.7 miles	1.1 to 1.4 miles	0.9 to 1.1 miles	Less than 0.9 mile
Females 30 to 39	Greater than 1.6 miles	1.2 to 1.6 miles	1.1 to 1.2 miles	0.9 to 1.1 miles	Less than 0.9 mile
Females 40 to 49	Greater than 1.4 miles	1.2 to 1.4 miles	0.9 to 1.2 miles	0.8 to 0.9 miles	Less than 0.8 mile
Females 50 and older	Greater than 1.4 miles	1.1 to 1.4 miles	0.9 to 1.1 miles	0.7 to 0.9 miles	Less than 0.7 mile

Table 13. Norms for twelve-minute walk/run aerobic fitness test

Source: Cooper.[1]

Appendix B
Submaximal Aerobic Fitness Test

Complete this test before beginning your six-week interval sprinting program. Set up your stationary bike as per the instructions in chapter 3 (page 80). The aim is to complete three bouts of continuous cycling for a total of ten minutes: four minutes, three minutes, and another three-minute stage. Record your heart rate and rating of perceived exertion (RPE) (see page 73) at the end of the three exercise stages. Typical heart rates should be around 100 beats per minute during stage one, 115 beats per minute during stage two, and 130 beats per minute during stage three for people in their twenties and thirties. For men and women in their forties and fifties, typical heart rates should be around 90 beats per minute during stage one, 105 beats per minute during stage two, and 120 beats per minute during stage three. For people in their sixties, heart rates should be about 80 beats per minute in stage one, 95 beats per minute in stage two, and 110 beats per minute in stage three. Your heart rate should not go above 140 beats per minute during the test.

Collect your data and then plot your heart-rate data on the graph in appendix C.

Male

Name:				Date:		
	Pedal rate	Pedal resistance	Heart rate	RPE		Collection time
Stage 1 4 minutes	60 rpm	2.2 pounds				At end of stage
Stage 2 3 minutes	60 rpm	3.3 pounds				At end of stage
Stage 3 3 minutes	60 rpm	4.4 pounds				At end of stage
Cool-down 4 minutes	40 rpm	1.1 pounds				

Female

Name:				Date:		
	Pedal rate	Pedal resistance	Heart rate	RPE		Collection time
Stage 1 4 minutes	60 rpm	1.1 pounds				At end of stage
Stage 2 3 minutes	60 rpm	2.2 pounds				At end of stage
Stage 3 3 minutes	60 rpm	4.4 pounds				At end of stage
Cool-down 4 minutes	40 rpm	1.1 pounds				

Appendix C
Monitoring Heart-Rate Change Using the Submaximal Fitness Test

If the submaximal test is repeated using the same workloads and under the same climatic conditions, the three heart rates at the three different pedal resistances will be lower if you have improved your aerobic fitness. Plotting your heart rates on this graph for a submaximal test repeated every three or four weeks should show a decrease in the heart-rate response. The decreased heart rate comes about because of increases in stroke volume and enhanced mitochondrial enzymes in the exercising muscles.

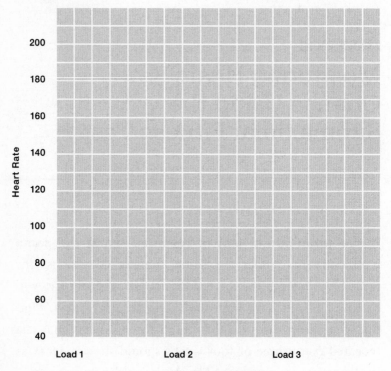

Appendix D
Rating of Perceived Exertion

We'd like you to use this scale to measure how your whole body feels during exercise, considering the total amount of exertion, and including all sensations of physical stress, effort, and fatigue in your body. If you feel no exertion at all, you would choose number 6, and if you feel maximum exertion, you would choose number 20. If you feel somewhere in between, then you would choose a number between 6 and 20. Remember, this scale refers to your *whole body* exertion, not your legs specifically. You can use any number from the scale to describe how you feel, which is likely to change during your exercise time.

Borg's RPE Scale

6	No exertion at all
7	Extremely light
8	
9	Very light
10	
11	Light
12	
13	Somewhat hard
14	
15	Hard (Heavy)
16	
17	Very hard
18	
19	Extremely hard
20	Maximal exertion

Appendix E
Body Composition Recording Form

This form contains variables that you can record weekly or twice weekly on a nonexercise day, allowing you to chart your progress to see which body composition variables change. Having someone else take the measures reduces error, and it is best if two measures are recorded and the average value documented. Instructions for collecting these measures can be found in chapter 1.

	Value 1	Value 2	Average
Name:			**Date:**
Session number:		**Time of day:**	**Temperature:**
Weight (pounds)			
Waist circumference (inches)			
Abdominal width (inches)			
Waist skinfold (inches; see pages 25-27)			
Upper leg circumference (inches)			
Lower leg circumference (inches)			

Comments:

Appendix F
Interval Sprinting Recording Form

This form contains variables that you can record before, during, and after each interval sprinting session. By recording these data, you can chart your progress to see if you improve. You can also use this information to adjust your pedal rate and pedal resistance as you increase your fitness and become accustomed to interval sprinting.

Name:					Date:	
Session number:			Time of day:		Temperature:	
Pre-exercise drink:			Water		Green tea	
	Pedal rate sprint	Pedal rate recovery	Pedal resistance	Heart rate	RPE	Collection time
Warm-up: 4 minutes						At end of warm-up
5 minutes						During 5th minute
10 minutes						During 10th minute
15 minutes						During 15th minute
20 minutes						During 20th minute
Cool-down: 4 minutes						During 24th minute

Comments:

Appendix G
Weekly Progress Form

This form contains variables that you can record sep-arately from the interval sprinting session, including body composition and cardiovascular data. Record your cholesterol, triglyceride, low-density lipoprotein (LDL), and high-density lipoprotein (HDL), and blood pressure levels, if you have them. Blood pressure is typically recorded as two numbers such as 120 over 80 millimeters of mercury (mmHg). Systolic blood pressure is the higher of the two numbers and measures the pressure in the arteries when the heart contracts, whereas diastolic blood pressure is the lower number and measures the artery pressure when the heart is resting. By recording these data, you can track any changes.

Name:		Date:		Time of day:	
Body composition		**Cardiovascular**		**Fitness, stress, sleep, fatigue, diet**	
Variable		**Variable**		**Variable**	
Weight		Resting heart rate		Submax test heart rate	
Body fat percentage		Systolic blood pressure		Stress levels	
Muscle mass		Diastolic blood pressure		Sleep quality	
Waist circumference		Cholesterol		Mediterranean eating score (see page 118)	
Waist skinfold		Trigs			
Abdominal width		LDL			
Midthigh circumference		HDL			
Lower leg circumference					
Comments:					

Acknowledgments

I would like to thank the many subjects in our studies who participated in these interval sprinting programs. Thanks also go to the many medical students who made a significant contribution to data collection. A team of PhD students organized and ran these studies, including Mehrdad Heydari, Ehsan Ghareman, and Sarah Dunn. The team at Black Inc. provided invaluable help that made this book possible. Finally, I would like to thank my wife, Yati, who made a significant contribution to the book, both from her published studies and with her editorial help and suggestions.

Resources

This section lists a number of useful books and web-sites that provide information for helping with lifestyle changes based on interval sprinting exercise and healthy eating.

Exercise

LifeSprints

LifeSprints is an interval sprinting music program based on the eight-second/twelve-second principle: sprinting for eight seconds followed by easy pedalling for twelve seconds. *LifeSprints* music is available on iTunes. The author has developed a website that includes lots of information regarding belly fat and up-to-date references on interval sprinting: www.bellyfatresearch.com.

Registered Clinical Exercise Physiologists (RCEPs)

In the USA the American College of Sports Medicine certifies health professionals called Registered Clinical Exercise Physiologists (RCEPs) who utilize scientific rationale to design, implement, and supervise exercise programming for individuals with chronic diseases and physical shortcomings. More information about RCEPs can be found at: http://certification .acsm.org.

BOOKS

McArdle, W. D., F. I. Katch, and V. L. Katch. *Exercise Physiology: Energy, Nutrition, and Human Performance*, 7th ed. Baltimore: Lippincott Williams & Wilkins, 2010. An excellent introductory text for exercise physiology.

Nutrition and Diet

BOOKS

Brand-Miller, J., et al. *Low GI Diet: 12-Week Weight-Loss Plan*. Sydney: Hachette Australia, 2012. This book contains useful information on glycemic index and diet.

Hyman, Mark. *UltraMetabolism: The Simple Plan for Automatic Weight Loss*. New York: Atria Books, 2006. This book provides an excellent overview of health and metabolism.

Tessmer, K., and S. Green. *The Complete Idiot's Guide to the Mediterranean Diet*. New York: Alpha Books, 2010. This book contains lots of Mediterranean recipes.

Wheeler, C., and D. A. Welland. *The Complete Idiot's Guide to Belly Fat Weight Loss*. New York: Alpha Books, 2012. This book contains useful information on diet and Mediterranean recipes.

WEBSITES

The National Weight Control Registry (www.nwcr.ws). The NWCR is a group of people who are monitored to help show what is most important for long-term weight control.

DietaryGuidelines.gov (www.health.gov/dietaryguidelines). This site provides evidence-based guidelines for lifestyle changes involving nutrition and physical activity.

Websites containing recipes and information on coconut: FreeCoconutRecipes.com (www.freecoconutrecipes.com) and Coconut Research Center (www.coconutresearchcenter.org).

Website containing information on protein in plants: Gentle World (www.gentleworld.org/10-protein-packed-plants).

Websites containing a range of Mediterranean recipes: EatingWell (www.eatingwell.com) and Allrecipes.com (www .allrecipes.com).

Stress Management

BOOKS

Borysenko, Joan. *Minding the Body, Mending the Mind.* Reading, MA: Addison-Wesley, 1987.

Davies, M., E. Eshelman, and M. McKay. *The Relaxation and Stress Reduction Workbook.* Oakland: New Harbinger, 2008.

Elkin, A. *Stress Management for Dummies.* New York: Alpha Books, 2013.

Seaward, Brian Luke. *Managing Stress: Principles and Strategies for Health and Well-Being.* Sudbury, MA: Jones and Bartlett, 2004.

WEBSITES

Three websites that contain a range of resources for dealing with stress: HelpGuide.org (www.helpguide.org); Mind Tools (www.mindtools.com); and the National Institute of Mental Health (www.nimh.nih.gov).

Sleep Quality

BOOKS AND ARTICLES

Espie, Colin. "How to Improve Your Sleep." *Guardian* (UK). January 29, 2011. www.guardian.co.uk/lifeandstyle/2011 /jan/29/how-to-improve-your-sleep.

Merrell, Woodson. *The Source*. New York: Free Press, 2000. A good overview of fatigue and energy and how they are related to sleep.

WEBSITES

WellnessMama.com, "How to Improve Your Sleep Naturally," www.wellnessmama.com/4936/how-to-improve-sleep -naturally.

Endnotes

Chapter 1: Understanding Belly Fat

1. K. M. Flegal, Carroll, M.D., Kit, B.K., and Ogden, C.L. "Prevalence of Obesity and Trends in the Distribution of Body Mass among US Adults, 1999-2010." *Journal of the American Medical Association* 307, no. 5 (February 2012): 491-97.

2. A. Misra, and L. Khurana, "Obesity and the Metabolic Syndrome in Developing Countries," *Journal of Clinical Endocrinology and Metabolism* 93, no. 11 (November 2008): S9–S30.

3. E. S. Ford et al., "Trends in Obesity and Abdominal Obesity Among Adults in the United States from 1999–2008," *International Journal of Obesity* 35, no. 5 (May 2011): 736–43.

4. E. J. Jacobs et al., "Waist Circumference and All-Cause Mortality in a Large US Cohort," *Archives of Internal Medicine* 170, no. 15 (August 9, 2011): 1293–301.

5. Children's Sizing Report Launch, *Shape GB: Measuring the Nation*, www.shapegb.org/childrens_sizing_report_launch.

6. B. L. Heitmann and P. Frederiksen, "Thigh Circumference and Risk of Heart Disease and Premature Death: Prospective Cohort Study," *British Medical Journal* 339 (2009): b3292, www.bmj.com/content/339/bmj.b3292.

7. K. L. Spalding et al., "Dynamics of Fat Cell Turnover in Humans," *Nature* 453, no. 7196 (June 5, 2008): 783–87.

8. B. L. Wajchenberg, "Subcutaneous and Visceral Adipose Tissue: Their Relation to the Metabolic Syndrome," *Endocrine Reviews* 21, no. 6 (December 2000): 697–738.

9. J. H. O'Keefe, K. A. Bybee, and C. J. Lavie, "Alcohol and Cardiovascular Health: The Razor-Sharp, Double-Edged Sword," *Journal of the American College of Cardiology* 50, no. 11 (September 11, 2007): 1009–14.

10. P. T. Katzmarzyk et al., "Racial Differences in Abdominal Depot-Specific Adiposity in White and African American Adults," *American Journal of Clinical Nutrition* 91, no. 1 (January 2010): 7–15.

11. J. P. Després et al., "Race, Visceral Adipose Tissue, Plasma Lipids, and Lipoprotein Lipase Activity in Men and Women: The Health, Risk Factors, Exercise Training, and Genetics (HERITAGE) Family Study," *Arteriosclerosis, Thrombosis, and Vascular Biology* 20, no. 8 (August 2000): 1932–38.

12. W. Y. Fujimoto et al., "Visceral Fat Obesity and Mortality: NIDDM and Atherogenic Risk in Japanese American Men and Women," supplement 2, *International Journal of Obesity* 15 (September 1991): 41–44.

13. M. A. Banerji et al., "Body Composition, Visceral Fat, Leptin, and Insulin Resistance in Asian Indian Men," *Journal of Clinical Endocrinology and Metabolism* 84, no. 1 (January 1999): 137–44.

14. S. S. Anand et al., "Adipocyte Hypertrophy, Fatty Liver and Metabolic Risk Factors in South Asians: The Molecular Study of Health and Risk in Ethnic Groups (mol-SHARE)," *PLoS ONE* 6, no. 7 (2011): e22112, doi:10.1371/journal.pone .0022112.

15. D. Canoy et al., "Cigarette Smoking and Fat Distribution in 21,828 British Men and Women: A Population-Based Study," *Obesity Research* 13, no. 8 (August 2005): 1466–75.

16. X. Hou et al., "Impact of Waist Circumference and Body Mass Index on Risk of Cardiometabolic Disorder and Cardiovascular Disease in Chinese Adults: A National Diabetes and Metabolic Disorders Survey," *PLoS ONE* 8, no. 3 (2013): e57319, doi:10.1371/journal.pone.0057319.

17. C. Raffaitin et al., "Metabolic Syndrome and Cognitive Decline in French Elders: The Three-City Study," *Neurology* 76, no. 6 (February 8, 2011): 518–25.

18. P. Guallar-Castillón et al., "Waist Circumference as a Predictor of Disability Among Older Adults," *Obesity* 15, no. 1 (2007): 233–44.

19. S. C. Larsson and A. Wolk, "Obesity and Colon and Rectal Cancer Risk: A Meta-Analysis of Prospective Studies," *American Journal of Clinical Nutrition* 86, no. 3 (September 2007): 556–65.

20. World Health Organization, "Appropriate Body-Mass Index for Asian Populations and Its Implications for Policy and Intervention Strategies," *Lancet* 363 no. 9403 (January 10, 2004): 157–63.

21. K. G. Alberti, P. Zimmet, and J. Shaw, "The Metabolic Syndrome—A New Worldwide Definition," *Lancet* 336, no. 9491 (September 24, 2005): 1059–62.

Chapter 2: The Effect of Exercise on Belly Fat and Health

1. T. Wu et al., "Long-Term Effectiveness of Diet-Plus-Exercise Interventions Vs. Diet-Only Interventions for Weight Loss: A Meta-Analysis," *Obesity Reviews* 10, no. 3 (May 2009): 313–23.

2. K. Ohkawara et al., "A Dose-Response Relation Between Aerobic Exercise and Visceral Fat Reduction: Systematic Review of Clinical Trials," *International Journal of Obesity* 31, no. 12 (December 2007): 1786–97.

3. I. Ismail et al., "A Systematic Review and Meta-Analysis of the Effect of Aerobic Vs. Resistance Exercise Training on Visceral Fat," *Obesity Reviews* 13, no. 1 (January 2013): 68–91.

4. A. Mourier et al., "Mobilization of Visceral Adipose Tissue Related to the Improvement in Insulin Sensitivity in Response to Physical Training in NIDDM. Effects of Branched-Chain Amino Acid Supplements," *Diabetes Care* 20, no. 3 (March 1997): 385–91.

5. E. G. Trapp et al., "The Effects of High-Intensity Intermittent Exercise Training on Fat Loss and Insulin Levels of Young Women," *International Journal of Obesity* 32, no. 4 (April 2008): 684–91.

6. S. L. Dunn, W. Siu, J. Freund, and S. H. Boutcher (in press), "The Effect of a Lifestyle Intervention on Metabolic Health in Young Women," *Diabetes, Metabolic Syndrome and Obesity: Targets and Therapy.*

7. M. Heydari, J. Freund, J, and S. H. Boutcher, "The Effect of High-Intensity Intermittent Exercise on Body Composition of Overweight Young Males," *Journal of Obesity* (2012): article ID 480467, doi:10.1155/2012/480467.

8. S. H. Boutcher, "High-Intensity Intermittent Exercise and Fat Loss," *Journal of Obesity* (2011): 868305. Epub 2010 Nov 24; Ohkawara et al., "A Dose-Response Relation"; Ismail et al., "Systematic Review and Meta-Analysis."

9. M. D. Peterson, A. Sen, and P. M. Gordon, "Influence of Resistance Exercise on Lean Body Mass in Aging Adults: A Meta-Analysis," *Medicine and Science in Sports and Exercise* 43, no. 2 (February 2011): 249–58.

10. Trapp et al., "Effects of High-Intensity Intermittent Exercise Training on Fat Loss and Insulin Levels"; Dunn, "Effects of Exercise and Dietary Intervention on Metabolic Syndrome Markers"; Heydari, Freund, and Boutcher, "Effect of High-Intensity Intermittent Exercise on Body Composition."

11. D. Thivel et al., "Intensive Exercise: A Remedy for Childhood Obesity?," *Physiology & Behavior* 102, no. 2 (February 1, 2011): 132–36.

12. M. Tan et al., "Effect of High-Intensity Intermittent Exercise on Plasma Postprandial Triacylglycerol in Sedentary Young Women," *International Journal of Sport Nutrition and Exercise Metabolism,* no. 24 (April 2014): 110–18.

13. S. H. Boutcher and S. L. Dunn, "Factors That May Impede the Weight Loss Response to Exercise-Based Interventions," *Obesity Reviews* 10, no. 6 (November 2009): 671–80.

14. Heydari, Freund, and Boutcher, "Effect of High-Intensity Intermittent Exercise on Body Composition."

15. S. N. Blair, "Physical Inactivity: The Biggest Public Health Problem of the 21st Century," *British Journal of Sports Medicine* 43, no. 1 (January 2009): 1-2.

16. Trapp et al., "Effects of High-Intensity Intermittent Exercise Training on Fat Loss and Insulin Levels."

17. Dunn, "Effects of Exercise and Dietary Intervention on Metabolic Syndrome Markers"; Heydari, Freund, and Boutcher, "Effect of High-Intensity Intermittent Exercise on Body Composition."

18. J. L. Kuk, P. M. Janiszewski, and R. Ross, "Exercise, Visceral Adipose Tissue, and Metabolic Risk," *Current Cardiovascular Risk Reports* 1, no. 3 (July 2007): 254–64; Trapp et al., "Effects of High-Intensity Intermittent Exercise Training on Fat Loss and Insulin Levels"; Dunn, "Effects of Exercise and Dietary Intervention on Metabolic Syndrome Markers."

19. K. Meyer et al., "Interval Training in Patients with Severe Chronic Heart Failure: Analysis and Recommendations for Exercise Procedures," *Medicine & Science in Sports and Exercise* 29, no. 3 (March 1997): 306–12.

20. P. S. Munk et al., "High-Intensity Interval Training May Reduce In-Stent Restenosis Following Percutaneous Coronary Intervention with Stent Implantation: A Randomized Controlled Trial Evaluating the Relationship to Endothelial Function and Inflammation," *American Heart Journal* 158, no. 5 (November 2009): 734–41.

21. T. T. Moholdt et al., "Aerobic Interval Training Versus Continuous Moderate Exercise After Coronary Artery Bypass Surgery: A Randomized Study of Cardiovascular Effects and Quality of Life," *American Heart Journal* 158, no. 6 (December 2009): 1031–37.

22. B. B. Nilsson, A. Westheim, and M. A. Risberg, "Long-Term Effects of a Group-Based High-Intensity Aerobic Interval Training Program in Patients with Chronic Heart Failure," *American Journal of Cardiology* 102, no. 9 (November 1, 2008): 1220–24.

23. U. Wisløff et al., "Superior Cardiovascular Effect of Aerobic Interval Training Versus Moderate Continuous Training in

Heart Failure Patients: A Randomized Study," *Circulation* 115, no. 24 (June 19, 2007): 3086–94.

24. Ø. Rognmo et al., "High Intensity Aerobic Interval Exercise Is Superior to Moderate Intensity Exercise for Increasing Aerobic Capacity in Patients with Coronary Artery Disease," *European Journal of Cardiovascular Prevention & Rehabilitation* 11, no. 3 (June 2004): 216–22.

25. C. Ernst, "The Role of Exercise Interval Training in Treating Cardiovascular Disease Risk Factors," *Current Cardiovascular Risk Reports* 3, no. 4 (July 2009): 296–301.

26. I. Vogiatzis et al., "Skeletal Muscle Adaptations to Interval Training with Patients with Advanced COPD," *CHEST* 128, no. 6 (December 2005): 3838–45.

27. Ibid.

28. E. A. Kortianou et al., "Effectiveness of Interval Exercise Training in Patients with COPD," *Cardiopulmonary Physical Therapy Journal* 21, no. 3 (September 2010): 12–19.

29. A. E. Tjønna et al., "Aerobic Interval Training Versus Continuous Moderate Exercise as a Treatment for the Metabolic Syndrome: A Pilot Study," *Circulation* 118, no. 4 (July 22, 2008): 346–54.

30. S. F. E. Praet et al., "Long-Standing, Insulin-Treated Type 2 Diabetes Patients with Complications Respond Well to Short-Term Resistance and Interval Exercise Training," *European Journal of Endocrinology* 158, no. 2 (February 2008): 163–72.

31. J. P. Little et al., "Low-Volume High-Intensity Interval Training Reduces Hyperglycemia and Increases Muscle Mitochondrial Capacity in Patients with Type 2 Diabetes," *Journal of Applied Physiology* 111, no. 6 (December 2011): 1554–60.

32. V. A. Bussau et al., "The 10-s Maximal Sprint: A Novel

Approach to Counter an Exercise-Mediated Fall in Glycemia in Individuals with Type 1 Diabetes," *Diabetes Care* 29, no. 3 (March 2006): 601–6.

33. K. J. Guelfi et al., "Effect of Intermittent High-Intensity Compared with Moderate Exercise on Glucose Production and Utilization in Individuals with Type 1 Diabetes," *American Journal of Physiology-Endocrinology and Metabolism* 292, no. 3 (March 2007): E865–70.

34. H. S. Kessler, S. B. Sisson, and K. R. Short, "The Potential for High-Intensity Interval Training to Reduce Cardiometabolic Disease Risk," *Sports Medicine* 42, no. 6 (June 1, 2012): 489–509.

35. S. A. Slørdahl et al., "Effective Training for Patients with Intermittent Claudication," *Scandinavian Cardiovascular Journal* 39, no. 4 (September 2005): 244–49.

36. J. Adams, "High-Intensity Interval Training for Intermittent Claudication in a Vascular Rehabilitation Program," *Journal of Vascular Nursing* 24, no. 2 (June 2006): 46–49.

37. Trapp et al., "Effects of High-Intensity Intermittent Exercise Training on Fat Loss and Insulin Levels"; Heydari, Freund, and Boutcher, "Effect of High-Intensity Intermittent Exercise on Body Composition."

38. R. H. Coker et al., "Influence of Exercise Intensity on Abdominal Fat and Adiponectin in Elderly Adults," *Metabolic Syndrome and Related Disorders* 7, no. 4 (August 2009): 363–68.

39. V. B. O'Leary et al.,"Exercise-Induced Reversal of Insulin Resistance in Obese Elderly Is Associated with Reduced Visceral Fat," *Journal of Applied Physiology* 100, no. 5 (May 2006): 1584–589.

40. A. E. Tjønna et al., "Aerobic Interval Training Reduces Cardiovascular Risk Factors More Than a Multi Treatment

Approach in Overweight Adolescents," *Clinical Science* 116, no. 4 (February 2009): 317–26.

41. Boutcher, "High-Intensity Intermittent Exercise."

42. Mourier et al., "Mobilization of Visceral Adipose Tissue."

43. Tjønna et al., "Aerobic Interval Training Versus Continuous Moderate Exercise."

Chapter 3: The Interval Sprinting Belly Fat Loss Program

1. R. M. Bracken, D. M. Linnane, and S. Brooks, "Plasma Catecholamine Responses to Brief Intermittent Maximal Intensity Exercise," *Amino Acids* 36, no. 2 (February 2009): 209–17.

2. E. G. Trapp, D. J. Chisholm, and S. H. Boutcher, "Metabolic Response of Trained and Untrained Women During High-Intensity Intermittent Cycle Exercise," *American Journal of Physiology* 293, no. 6 (December 2007): R2370–R75.

3. R. J. Robertson, *Perceived Exertion for Practitioners: Rating Effort with the OMNI Picture System* (Champaign, IL: Human Kinetics, 2004).

4. M. Heydari and S. H. Boutcher, "Rating of Perceived Exertion After 12 Weeks of High-Intensity Intermittent Sprinting," *Perceptual & Motor Skills* 116, no. 1 (February 2013): 340–51.

5. Trapp, Chisholm, and Boutcher, "Metabolic Response of Trained and Untrained Women."

6. Ibid.

7. Bracken, Linnane, and Brooks, "Plasma Catecholamine Responses."

8. M. E. Nevill et al., "Growth Hormone Responses to Treadmill Sprinting in Sprint- and Endurance-Trained Athletes,"

European Journal of Applied Physiology and Occupational Physiology 72, nos. 5/6 (March 1996): 460–67.

Chapter 4: Dieting, Nutrients, and Belly Fat

1. J. H. O'Keefe and L. Cordain, "Cardiovascular Disease Resulting from a Diet and Lifestyle at Odds with Our Paleolithic Genome: How to Become a 21st-Century Hunter-Gatherer," *Mayo Clinic Proceedings* 79, no. 1 (January 2004): 101–8.

2. www.freecoconutrecipes.com; www.coconutresearchcenter.org.

3. M. M. Engler and M. B. Engler, "Omega-3 Fatty Acids: Role in Cardiovascular Health and Disease," *Journal of Cardiovascular Nursing* 21, no. 1 (January/February 2006): 17–24.

4. T. C. Campbell and T. M. Campbell, *The China Study: The Most Comprehensive Study of Nutrition Ever Conducted and the Startling Implications for Diet, Weight Loss, and Long-Term Health* (Dallas: BenBella Books, 2006).

5. www.gentleworld.org/10-protein-packed-plants.

6. B. Fife, *Saturated Fat May Save Your Life* (Colorado Springs, CO: Piccadilly Books, 1999).

7. R. Micha, S. K. Wallace, and D. Mozaffarian, "Red and Processed Meat Consumption and Risk of Incident Coronary Heart Disease, Stroke, and Diabetes Mellitus: A Systematic Review and Meta-Analysis," *Circulation* 121, no. 21 (June 1, 2010): 2271–83.

8. www.gentleworld.org/10-protein-packed-plants.

9. T. Mann et al., "Medicare's Search for Effective Obesity Treatments: Diets Are Not the Answer," *American Psychologist* 62, no. 3 (April 2007): 220–33.

10. T. B. Chaston and J. B. Dixon, "Factors Associated with Percent

Change in Visceral Versus Subcutaneous Abdominal Fat During Weight Loss: Findings from a Systematic Review," *International Journal of Obesity* 32, no. 4 (April 2008): 619–28.

11. M. de Lorgeril, "Mediterranean Diet in the Prevention of Coronary Heart Disease," *Nutrition* 14, no. 1 (January 1998): 55–57.

12. M. de Lorgeril and P. Salen, "The Mediterranean-Style Diet for the Prevention of Cardiovascular Diseases," *Public Health Nutrition* 9, no. 1A (February 2006): 118–23.

13. A. Trichopoulou et al., "Adherence to a Mediterranean Diet and Survival in a Greek Population," *New England Journal of Medicine* 348, no. 26 (June 26, 2003): 2599–608.

14. J. H. O'Keefe, K. A. Bybee, and C. J. Lavie, "Alcohol and Cardiovascular Health: The Razor-Sharp, Double-Edged Sword," *Journal of the American College of Cardiology* 50, no. 11 (September 11, 2007): 1009–14.

15. A. G. Tsai and T. A. Wadden, "Systematic Review: An Evaluation of Major Commercial Weight Loss Programs in the United States," *Annals of Internal Medicine* 142, no. 1 (January 4, 2005): 56–66.

16. M. L. Klem et al., "A Descriptive Study of Individuals Successful at Long-Term Maintenance of Substantial Weight Loss," *American Journal of Clinical Nutrition* 66, no. 2 (August 1997): 239–46.

17. T. F. Hsu et al., "Polyphenol-Enriched Oolong Tea Increases Fecal Lipid Excretion," *European Journal of Clinical Nutrition* 60, no. 11 (November 2006): 1330–36.

18. E. Bravo, M. Napolitano, and K. Botham, "Postprandial Lipid Metabolism: The Missing Link Between Life-Style Habits and the Increasing Incidence of Metabolic Diseases in Western Countries?," *Open Translational Medicine Journal* 2 (2010): 1–13.

19. Tan et al., "Effect of High-Intensity Intermittent Exercise on Plasma Postprandial Triacylglycerol."

20. J. H. O'Keefe, N. M. Gheewala, and J. O. O'Keefe, "Dietary Strategies for Improving Post-Prandial Glucose, Lipids, Inflammation, and Cardiovascular Health," *Journal of the American College of Cardiology* 51, no. 3 (January 2008): 249–55.

21. E. Ghahramanloo, "Effects of Green Tea Extract and High Intensity Intermittent Exercise on Fat Metabolism" (doctoral dissertation, University of New South Wales, 2012), http://unswroks .unsw.edu.au/vital/access/manager/Repository/unsworks: 345.

22. M. C. Venables et al., "Green Tea Extract Ingestion, Fat Oxidation, and Glucose Tolerance in Healthy Humans," *American Journal of Clinical Nutrition* 87, no. 3 (March 2008): 778–84.

23. K. Van Proeyen et al., "Training in the Fasted State Improves Glucose Tolerance During Fat-Rich Diet," *Journal of Physiology* 588, pt. 21 (November 1, 2010): 4289–302.

24. C. Martins et al., "Effects of Exercise on Gut Peptides, Energy Intake and Appetite," *Journal of Endocrinology* 193, no. 2 (May 2007): 251–58.

25. A. Y. Sim et al., "High-Intensity Intermittent Exercise Attenuates Ad-Libitum Energy Intake," *International Journal of Obesity* (June 4, 2013): doi:10.1038/ijo. Epub ahead of print.

26. L. J. White et al., "Increased Caloric Intake Soon After Exercise in Cold Water," *International Journal of Sport Nutrition and Exercise Metabolism* 15, no. 1 (February 2005): 38–47.

Chapter 5: Reducing Daily Stress and Enhancing Sleep Quality

1. J. Borysenko, *Minding the Body, Mending the Mind* (Reading, MA: Addison-Wesley, 1987).

2. K. Forcier et al., "Links Between Physical Fitness and Cardiovascular Reactivity and Recovery to Psychological Stressors: A Meta-Analysis," *Health Psychology* 25, no. 6 (November 2006): 723–39.

3. Trapp et al. "Metabolic Response of Trained and Untrained Women During High-Intensity, Intermittent exercise."

4. M. Heydari, Boutcher Y. N., and Boutcher S. H. "High-Intensity Intermittent Exercise and Cardiovascular and Autonomic function," *Journal of Clinical Autonomic Function* 23, no. 1 (2013), 57–65.

5. M. Heydari, Boutcher Y. N., and Boutcher S. H. "The Effects of High-Intensity Intermittent Exercise Training on Cardiovascular Response to Mental and Physical Challenge," *International Journal of Psychophysiology* 87, no. 2 (2013): 141–46.

6. S. R. Patel and F. B. Hu, "Short Sleep Duration and Weight Gain: A Systematic Review," *Obesity* 16, no. 3 (March 2008): 643–53.

7. K. G. Hairston et al., "Sleep Duration and Five-Year Abdominal Fat Accumulation in a Minority Cohort: The IRAS Family Study," *Sleep* 33, no. 3 (March 2010): 289–95.

Chapter 6: A Six-Week Belly Fat Loss Program

1. Fish tacos with avocado salsa recipe: www.taste.com.au/recipes/16763/fish+tacos+with+avocado+salsa.

2. Tahini tuna salad recipe: www.mamavation.com/2012/03/tahini-tuna-salad.html.

3. Garden vegetable wrap recipe: www.spryliving.com/recipes/garden-vegetable-wrap.

4. Black bean salad recipe: www.simplyrecipes.com/ingredients /black_bean/

5. Satay chicken with steamed vegetables recipe: www.taste.com .au/recipes/10415/satay+chicken+with+steamed+vegetables.

6. Shrimp and vegetable quinoa fried rice recipe: www.queen ofquinoa.me/2012/09/shrimp-vegetable-quinoa-fried-rice.

7. Tandoori chicken with fresh vegetables and rice recipe: www .sbs.com.au/food/recipe/121/Tandoori-chicken.

8. Grilled halibut with avocado and chipotle cream sauce recipe: www.avocadocentral.com/avocado-recipes/Grilled-Halibut -with-Avocado-Chipotle-Cream-Sauce.

9. Vegetable steak stir-fry recipe: www.tasteofhome.com/recipes /Vegetable-Steak-Stir-Fry.

10. Cod poached in tomato sauce with spinach, capers, and pine nuts recipe: www.thescrumptiouspumpkin.com/2012/11/02 /cod-poached-in-tomato-sauce-with-spinach-capers-and-pine -nuts.

11. Trapp et al., "Effects of High-Intensity Intermittent Exercise Training on Fat Loss and Insulin Levels"; Dunn, "Effects of Exercise and Dietary Intervention on Metabolic Syndrome Markers"; Boutcher, "High-Intensity Intermittent Exercise."

Appendix A

1. K. H. Cooper, "A Means of Assessing Maximal Oxygen Uptake: Correlation Between Field and Treadmill Testing," *Journal of the American Medical Association* 203, no. 3 (January 15, 1968): 201–4.

Index

Index

Index

Index

University of New South Wales: interval
sprinting studies at, 2, 36–37
University of Pittsburgh: sleep study at, 169
University of South Carolina: aerobic
fitness studies at, 46–47
unsaturated fats, 104, 106, 122, 124, 125
upper body: interval sprinting and,
94–95, 175, 176
upper legs: circumference of, 28, 97,
181, 192, 196

vegetable oils, 103, 106, 108
vegetables
and effects of nutrients on fat
burning, 139
and fat and sugar in blood after
eating meals, 142
frozen, 125
and Mediterranean eating plan,
115, 116, 118, 121, 124–26,
128, 130–31, 133–34, 178
pesticides and, 121–22
and processed food, 106, 109, 110,
111, 112
questionnaire about, 105
and reasons for becoming
overweight, 104
vegetarian diet, 111
visceral fat. *See* belly fat
vitamin A, 120, 124
vitamin B, 115
vitamin C, 120, 121, 124, 134, 140
vitamin E, 140
vitamins, 113, 114, 120, 122. *See also*
specific vitamin

waist circumference
aerobic exercise and, 38
average, 6
BMI and, 24
cancer and, 20
criteria for, 23
and effects of interval sprinting on
belly fat, 36, 37, 38, 46, 173
effects of interval sprinting on,
27–28, 35–36
ethnicity and, 19, 23, 24
and factors in accumulation of
belly fat, 11
gender and, 23, 24
health effects of, 19, 20, 24
increase in, 5–6
measurement of, 24, 25, 29
recording information about, 97,
181, 192, 196
resistance exercise and, 38

waist skinfold. *See* skinfold measurement
walking, 32, 59, 63, 92, 93, 159
warm-up, 88
water
cold, 145
and effects of dieting on belly fat,
113–14
and effects of exercise on appetite,
145
and effects of nutrients on belly fat,
136–37
and interval sprinting program, 88,
100–101, 176, 180
and measurement of belly fat, 23
Mediterranean eating plan and,
119, 126, 132, 178
recording information about, 194
weekly progress recording form, 195–96
weight
and age, 166
BMI and, 21–22
classification of, 22
dieting and, 113–14
and effects of belly fat on health, 19
and measuring sweat loss, 79
and monitoring progress, 96
pregnancy and, 64
recording information about, 96,
100, 101, 176, 181, 196
and six-week belly fat loss
program, 176, 181
sleep and, 165, 166, 168–69
stress and, 163
weight lifting, 42
weight training, 2, 14, 34, 41
Welland, Diane A., 126
Wheeler, Claire, 126
whole body exertion: measurement of,
189–90
whole foods, 139
whole grains, 109, 115, 125, 126–27,
133
wine. *See* alcohol
Wingate test, 34–35, 70, 75, 77
women
and accumulation of belly fat, 14, 63
ethnicity of, 14
increase in obesity in, 5
waist circumference for, 5–6
See also gender; postmenopausal
women; postpregnant women
work: stress at, 159–60

X-ray, 36. *See also* DEXA

yogurt, 115, 120, 127, 128, 133, 178